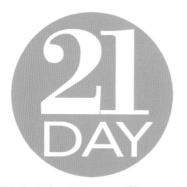

21 DAY METABOLISM makeover™

D1320084

3 Weeks of Simple Tweaks
That Will Turn Your Body
Into a **Fat Burning Machine!**

WHAT IS THE
METABOLISM MAKEOVER?

21 Days That Will Change Your Body... And Your Life!

The **21 Day Metabolism Makeover** is essentially a three week "induction" phase designed to "jump start" a metabolism slowed by age, repeated "yoyo" or "starvation" dieting, or by eating habits that have thrown your body into "Fat Storing Mode" and have kept it there. During this 21-day induction phase you'll learn how to make a few simple changes that will **optimize** your body's natural processes so that **it burns more of the calories you eat for energy and stores less of them as fat**.

Little Changes That Give You HUGE Results

This first 21 days is the only portion of the **Food Lovers** program with any real hard and fast "rules." By choosing the very best fat burning foods and avoiding, for this brief period, those most likely to slow your metabolism you will switch your body from "Fat Storing Mode" to "Fat Burning Mode" and literally *turn your body into a Fat Burning Machine all in just three weeks time!*

But even during this induction phase, we make it easy. You don't have to overhaul your lifestyle. **You only make one or two small changes a day**. And the best part is, you'll see for yourself how making just a few small changes can give you HUGE results.

Over the next three weeks you will "reset" your sluggish metabolism, shifting it into high gear, and causing your body to shed pounds and inches fast. Then you'll be ready to move on to the **Food Lovers for Life** program where the rules loosen up again. And, with your metabolism now converting calories to energy so quickly, *you'll be able to eat literally ALL your favorite foods in a way that will cause you to lose weight rather than gain it.*

The Key to Lasting Weight Loss

The **21 Day Metabolism Makeover** isn't just a quick way to lose a lot of fat. *It also makes it easy to keep the fat off.* Sure, there are lots of programs that can help you lose pounds quickly… for a short period of time. You could go on one of the numerous fad diets – perhaps eat only prepackaged foods that are sent to you in the mail each month or drink nothing but canned weight loss shakes – and you might lose some weight.

But what happens *after* you lose the weight? Are you really going to eat nothing but freeze-dried foods and canned shakes for the rest of your life? Of course not. You'll likely go back to the way you used to eat and gain all the weight back… probably more.

The problem with quick-fix programs like those is **they don't TEACH you anything about HOW to eat to be lean**. If you want to lose weight and KEEP IT OFF, you need to learn how to eat real food in the real world in a way that causes you to lose weight rather than gain it.

How to Be Lean For a Lifetime

As the old saying goes, "***Give a man a fish, you feed him for a day. Teach a man to fish, you feed him for a lifetime***." Well, the same holds true for weight loss. If you give a person a diet, he or she may lose weight for a week or two, but if you **teach that person how to eat in a way that causes them to lose weight, they'll be lean for a lifetime**.

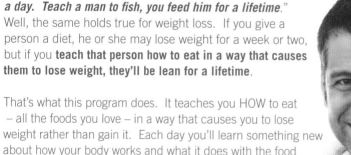

That's what this program does. It teaches you HOW to eat – all the foods you love – in a way that causes you to lose weight rather than gain it. Each day you'll learn something new about how your body works and what it does with the food you put into it. You'll learn the simple science that will make weight loss easy.

Get Started Today

Everything you need to lose all the weight you want and keep it off for the rest of your life is in your hands right now. So don't wait another minute. Turn the page and get started today. **The next 21 days will truly change your body… and your life!**

BEFORE YOU START...

① Watch the Quick Start DVD

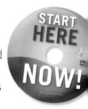

Before you do anything else, pop in the **Quick Start DVD** if you haven't already. In it, we'll walk you through everything you need to know to get started fast. We'll show you how to use each piece of the program and share tips for maximizing your success on the program. **This is where you start!**

② Read and Complete the Rapid Results Success Journal

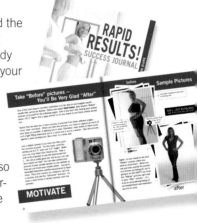

Before you start Day 1 of the program, read the **Rapid Results Success Journal** and fill it out **completely**. Do all the steps. Take your body measurements and "Before" pictures. Do your Body Composition Analysis and fill in the goal setting and self-assessment sections. You may be tempted to skip this and jump right into the program but don't! **This step is critical to your success.** In the back of the **Rapid Results Success Journal**, you'll also find a **Troubleshooting Guide** to help accelerate your results if you don't feel like you are getting results as fast as you should.

③ Fill in Your Planner Pages with Appointments for the Next 3 Weeks

The **21 Day Metabolism Makeover** is designed as a Daily Planner. In it you'll find Planner Pages with spaces to schedule all your appointments as well as sections to keep track of calls and daily tasks so, once your **Food Lovers** binder is put together, it will contain everything you need to lose all the weight you want – PLUS, it will function as your Daily Planner and To Do List, all in one easy-to-reference binder. Using your Food Lovers binder as your datebook will encourage you to keep it with you at all times and help assure your success! So, get out your family's calendar, appointment book or cell phone – whatever you keep your personal schedule in – and copy the next three week's worth of appointments into the Planner Pages of your **21 Day Metabolism Makeover**.

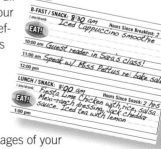

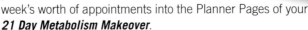

THE FAST TRACK
An Alternate Approach

The *21 Day Metabolism Makeover* is designed to make getting started on the **Food Lovers** program super-easy – you just take one small baby-step each day for 21 days.   However, if you prefer to dive right in and go full-bore right from the beginning, that's fine too. Here's what you do: all the significant changes to the way you are eating happen in the first 7 days, so simply read Days 1 to 7 and listen to the audio programs that correspond with those days. They can be found on the Fat Loss Secrets Day-By-Day audio series CDs. Also read the *How to Make a Fat Loss Plate* booklet. Then on the first day of your *21 Day Metabolism Makeover*, begin eating according to the guidelines given in those materials. And because you've jumped ahead by one full week, you'll begin your *21 Day Metabolism Makeover* by reading Day 8 and following the directions for that day. On your second day, read and do Day 9, and so on. When you get to Day 20 (which will actually be your 13th Day on the *21 Day Metabolism Makeover*), just continue doing what you're doing for an extra 7 days to make sure you have completely reset your metabolism. Then on the 21st Day of your *21 Day Metabolism Makeover*, read Day 21 and do the activities described. After that, you're ready to proceed to *Food Lovers for Life*.

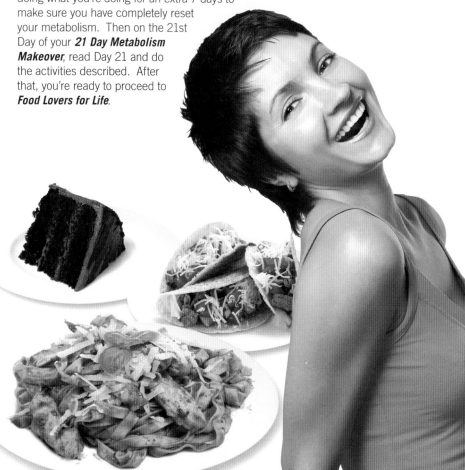

YOUR EATING JOURNAL
A CRITICAL KEY TO YOUR SUCCESS

In addition to being a powerful appointment calendar, your *21 Day Metabolism Makeover* is an "Eating Journal" where you'll keep track of what you eat and drink on each day of the program. **Daily journaling is an indispensable part of Food Lovers** that is critical for your success!

Within the Planner Pages are boxes for you to write down what you eat at each meal or snack. You'll find specific instructions for how to fill these sections out on the next page but the critically important thing is that you **write down EVERYTHING you eat and drink!**

SIMPLE SECRETS TO SUCCESS
Studies have shown that people who consistently keep a detailed daily eating journal eat 26% less food, **lose 64% more weight and keep the weight off** longer than those who do not!

And that means *everything*: every french fry nabbed off your spouse's plate, every piece of candy you grab from the bowl at the office, every sip you steal of your kid's soda. No matter how insignificant it may seem, **it will help you to write down everything you put in your mouth**. The more diligent and detailed you are, the more successful you'll be. It's also important to record "when" you eat, as well as "how long" it's been since you last ate, because regular eating is critical to speeding up your metabolism and increasing the rate that you burn fat.

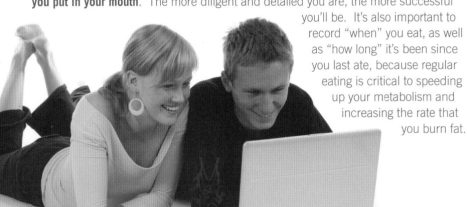

As you get into some of the later days in your *21 Day Metabolism Makeover*, you'll begin to record other activities which can have an effect on fat loss. You'll keep records of what exercise you do, how many hours you sleep at night, what nutritional supplements such as vitamins and minerals you take each day, and even how you "feel" each day.

This journal will be an invaluable asset to you. **Take the time, every day, to fill out the information required… in detail**. When you have a "great" week and shed a lot of body fat, you'll be able to look back and see exactly what you did that caused your body to lose the weight. When you have a week with less results, again you'll be able to consult your journal to determine exactly what it was that slowed your progress.

Often times you'll be surprised by the results. The key piece of information – the specific meal or variation in your eating schedule that increased or decreased your results – may be unapparent to you until you review your journal. This journal will reveal a wealth of information about how your body works – information that will allow you to maximize your results and learn how to be lean and healthy for the rest of your life.

Remember, **this is your journal, so be honest**. If you slip up, don't beat yourself up. Just describe how and why it happened in the "Notes" section of the Planner Pages so that you learn from the experience and get right back on track.

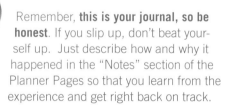

Those who are diligent about journaling succeed, and those who don't, DON'T!

HOW TO USE YOUR PLANNER PAGES

A Fill in the date and day of the week.

B Today's Activity - The section tells you the simple tweaks you are making today in order to speed up your metabolism.

C The "To Do List" contains a comprehensive list of everything you should be doing on this day. Check them off as you complete them. Use the blank spaces for your own personal tasks for the day. (Call Stan, Sign Kids Up for Soccer, Pay Water Bill, etc.)

D Eating Times - Keep track of your eating schedule by filling in the time you ate your meal or snack as well as the amount of time since you ate last in these spaces.

E Eating Journal - Next to each colored plate write down everything you ate or drank at each meal or snack. Be as detailed as possible including quantities, portion sizes, ingredients, beverages, condiments, sweeteners, bites tasted from another person's plate, EVERYTHING!

F Planner Pages - You're going to carry this with you wherever you go. So use this as your appointment book and copy all your appointments for the next three weeks into the pages.

G Exercise - If you do any exercise on a given day, write down the details of your routine.

DAY 1

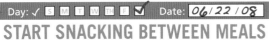

Day: ✓ S M T W TH F ✓ **Date:** 06/22/08

START SNACKING BETWEEN MEALS

Today you are going to simply start snacking! Add a snack between each meal every 2 to 3 hours and in the evening until one hour before bed. Ideally, you'll choose snacks from the **Snack & Treat Guide**, but the most important thing is that you eat a meal or snack every 2 to 3 hours to speed up your metabolism so you burn more fat.

TO DOS
(check when done)

- ☑ Read & complete **Rapid Results Success Journal**
- ☑ Listen to the **Day 1** Audio Program
- ☑ Eat every 2 to 3 hours
- ☑ Write down EVERYTHING I put in my mouth today
- ☑ Read pages X to X of **How to Make a Fat Loss Plate**
- ☑ ~~Tomorrow's Fat~~ Plate
- ☑ Pick Up Dry Cleaning
- ☑ Get Gift ~~for~~ Sus~~ie~~
- ☐ _____
- ☐ _____
- ☐ _____
- ☐ _____

TODAY'S CALLS

_____
_____
_____
_____
_____
_____

TODAY'S SCHEDULE

B-FAST / SNACK: 7:00 am **Mins. Since Waking Up:** 5 min
I ate/drank: Tuscan Omelet
Decaf Coffee (black)
EAT!

7:00 am

8:00 am — Morning walk

9:00 am

B-FAST / SNACK: 9:30 am **Hours Since Breakfast:** 2½ hrs
I ate/drank: Two Food Lovers Oatmeal Raisin Cookies
Sparkling Water w/ Lime
EAT!

10:00 am

11:00 am — Take Sparky to vet

__:__ pm

LUNCH / SNACK: 12:30 **Hours Since Snack:** 3 hrs
I ate/drank: Chicken Sandwich w/ Lettuce, Tomatoes, & Mustard
Side Salad (Field Greens, Cherry Tomatoes, Carrots, & 2 TBSP Balsamic Vinaigrette Dressing)
Iced Tea w/ Lemon
EAT!

1:00 pm

2:00 pm

SNACK: 3:00 **Hours Since Lunch:** 2½ hrs
I ate/drank: Food Lovers Blueberry Muffin
Glass of water
EAT!

EXERCISE ☑ YES ☐ NO **TIME** 45 min
What/how much? 45 minutes of walking
30 Situps

THE FOOD LOVERS FAT LOSS SYSTEM

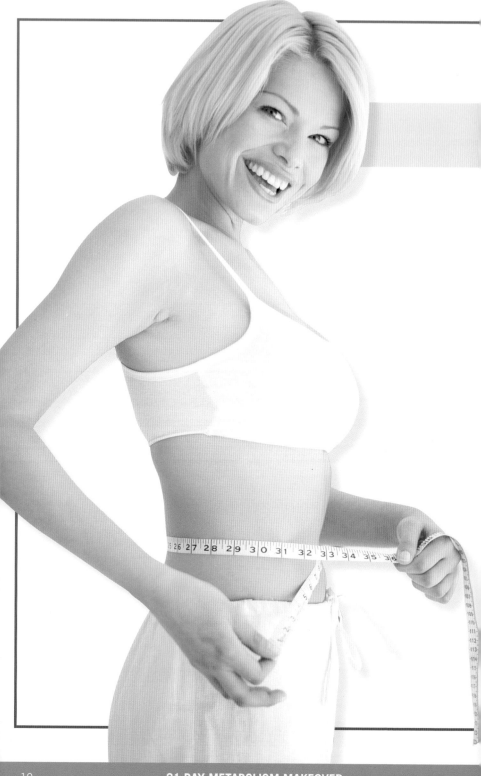

21 DAY METABOLISM MAKEOVER

THAT'S IT.
YOU'RE READY TO GO!

So turn the page and begin creating the lean healthy body you deserve.

The next 21 Days really can
change your body...
And your life!

Before starting this or any other fat loss program, please consult with your physician.

TODAY we start to **USE FOOD TO BURN FAT!** 21 days from now, you will have completely made over your metabolism and then, **YOU'LL NEVER HAVE TO DIET AGAIN!**

DAY 1:
START SNACKING
BETWEEN MEALS

Today you are going to begin to jump start your metabolism by adding snacks between the meals you normally eat over the course of the day. **Eat a snack about midway between Breakfast and Lunch, and another one between Lunch and Dinner. Then, after Dinner keep eating a snack every 2 to 3 hours until one hour before you go to bed.** For today, it can be whatever you want: a couple handfuls of potato chips, an apple, a half-sandwich, whatever sounds good. Just make sure you **write down every single thing you eat and drink** today along with when you eat them in the following Planner Pages.

How Will Eating MORE
Help Me Lose Weight?

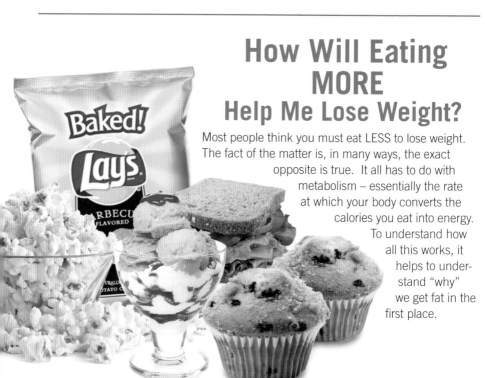

Most people think you must eat LESS to lose weight. The fact of the matter is, in many ways, the exact opposite is true. It all has to do with metabolism – essentially the rate at which your body converts the calories you eat into energy. To understand how all this works, it helps to understand "why" we get fat in the first place.

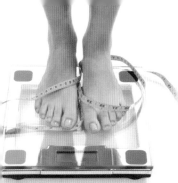

Why We Get Fat

For most of mankind's history food has been scarce - and most of our days were spent hunting, gathering and basically trying to keep ourselves from starving to death. To help keep us alive, biology came up with an ingenious survival strategy: when food was running low, our bodies would *slow down our metabolism*. It would start burning less calories for energy and instead it would save them for later use… by **storing them as fat**. It worked great when food was hard to come by but now that food is plentiful and a fast food lunch can easily contain 1500 calories - a full days calories for most people - it's not so great.

Why Diets Don't Work

While our body's super-efficient ability to store calories (energy) as fat has helped mankind survive through the ages, this really becomes a problem when you go on a diet. That's because when you start dieting and cut way back on calories or go a long time without eating, your body doesn't know you are "dieting." **It thinks you are actually starving.** It says to itself, "I don't know when I'll eat again, so I'd better store as many calories as I can (as fat!), instead of burning it as fuel, so I'll have it later and not die of starvation." It goes into "survival mode" and slows your metabolism. **So, even though you are eating less food, your body stores more of it as fat.**

If you've ever dieted, you may have experienced this. After a few weeks of extreme dieting your weight loss slows - then stops. You may begin to gain weight even though you are practically eating nothing. That is because you've essentially **"shut down" your metabolism**. Even worse, when you finally fall off the starvation diet – and we all do at some point because nobody can keep that up for long -- your metabolism will be so slow that eating just "regular" food again will not only cause you to regain the weight you lost, but, *often, put on even more!*

Turn Your Metabolism Around

With the **Food Lovers** program, you'll reverse this starving and gaining cycle and start **eating** and **losing** instead. **By eating more often throughout the day, you will actually speed up your metabolism, which in turn will help you burn off excess body fat. The key is to eat EVERY 2 to 3 hours, all day long.** This regularly scheduled intake of food lets your body know that there will always be plenty of fuel to burn, that there is no need to worry about starving to death and that it can stop storing so many calories as fat.

It may seem like a small first step, but just by starting to eat at regular intervals you're not only speeding up your metabolism, but you've begun to undo the damage done by years of dieting. You'll find that you have more energy, that you've reduced the cravings and hunger that cause you to overeat, and that you are now eating in a way that helps you retain lean muscle tissue which will eventually cause you to burn more calories all day long.

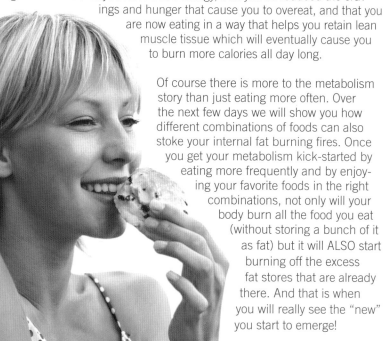

Of course there is more to the metabolism story than just eating more often. Over the next few days we will show you how different combinations of foods can also stoke your internal fat burning fires. Once you get your metabolism kick-started by eating more frequently and by enjoying your favorite foods in the right combinations, not only will your body burn all the food you eat (without storing a bunch of it as fat) but it will ALSO start burning off the excess fat stores that are already there. And that is when you will really see the "new" you start to emerge!

WHAT TO SNACK ON

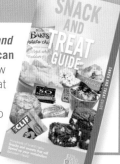

You'll find more than 1000 great tasting snacks in the *Snack and Treat Guide* - including more than 100 sweet treats - that you can make or find in any grocery or convenience store. The first few pages will show you how to choose the very best snacks for fat loss, but for today just eat anything you feel like eating. The key is to let your body know that it isn't going to be starving so it starts to move into "Fat Burning Mode."

DO THIS TODAY

① Start Snacking Between Meals
The most important change you are going to make today is to start snacking between meals. Add a snack between Breakfast and Lunch, Lunch and Dinner and every 2 to 3 hours in the evening until an hour before going to bed to speed up your metabolism. **Never go more than three hours without eating!**

② Starting Today, Write Down Everything You Eat
Studies have shown that people who consistently keep a detailed daily eating journal lose 64% more weight than those who do not. *And they keep the weight off longer.* Next to each colored plate on the Planner Pages, write down everything you eat and drink – no matter how small – and **note the time you started to eat each meal and snack.**

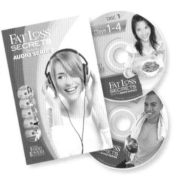

③ Listen to Day 1 of the Fat Loss Secrets CD
These pages are just the start. In this powerful audio program, we will give you the knowledge to take your metabolism to the next level. **Pick a time and make sure you listen to the audios on each and every one of your 21 days**. Start your day listening at home or pop it in the car while driving to work. As you will quickly discover, the audio CD is going to be like having a personal chef, private trainer and full time motivator with you making sure you get the results you want.

④ Get Ready for Tomorrow
Starting tomorrow you are going to begin to switch your body from "Fat Storing Mode" to "Fat Burning Mode" by eating a **Food Lovers Fat Loss Plate** for Lunch or Dinner. To make sure you are ready, read through pages 1 to 29 in *How to Make a Fat Loss Plate* tonight, decide whether your Fat Loss Plate is going to be Lunch or Dinner and also read the section for the meal you've chosen, then make sure you have the foods you need to make your meal. If you want to learn more about the science behind the Fat Loss Plate, you can continue on to the section entitled "Why it Works" which begins on page 30.

Congratulations! You've taken the first step towards re-setting your metabolism and turning your body into a fat burning machine!
Tomorrow you'll learn how to use the right combinations of your favorite foods to switch your body to "Fat Burning Mode".

DAY 1

START SNACKING BETWEEN MEALS

Today you are going to simply start snacking! Add a snack between each meal and every 2 to 3 hours in the evening until one hour before bed. Ideally, you'll choose snacks from the **Snack & Treat Guide**, but the most important thing is that you eat a meal or snack every 2 to 3 hours to spe up your metabolism so you burn more fat.

✓ TO DOS
(check when done)

- ☐ Read & Complete **Rapid Results Success Journal**
- ☐ Listen to the **Day 1** Audio Program
- ☐ Eat every 2 to 3 hours
- ☐ Write down EVERYTHING I put in my mouth today
- ☐ Read pages 1 to 29 of **How to Make a Fat Loss Plate**
- ☐ Plan tomorrow's Fat Loss Plate
- ☐ _____
- ☐ _____
- ☐ _____
- ☐ _____

TODAY'S CALLS

_____
_____
_____
_____
_____
_____
_____
_____

TODAY'S SCHEDULE

B-FAST / SNACK: Time _____   **Mins. Since Waking Up:** Time _____

I ate/drank:

EAT!

_____
7:00 am
_____
8:00 am
_____
9:00 am
_____

B-FAST / SNACK: Time _____   **Hours Since Breakfast:** Time _____

I ate/drank:

EAT!

_____
10:00 am
_____
11:00 am
_____
12:00 pm
_____

LUNCH / SNACK: Time _____   **Hours Since Snack:** Time _____

I ate/drank:

EAT!

_____
1:00 pm
_____
2:00 pm
_____

SNACK: Time _____   **Hours Since Lunch:** Time _____

I ate/drank:

EAT!

EXERCISE   ☐ YES   ☐ NO   **TIME** [_____]

What/how much?
_____
_____

THE PERFECT FAT LOSS SNACK

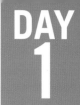

DAY 1

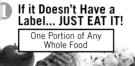

1 **If it Doesn't Have a Label... JUST EAT IT!**

One Portion of Any Whole Food

2 **If it *Has* a Label...**
Anything you want as long as it's:

Men & Women:
150 - 250 Calories

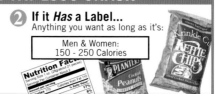

TODAY'S SCHEDULE

3:00 pm

4:00 pm

5:00 pm

NNER: Time   **Hours Since Snack:** Time

te/drank:

EAT!

6:00 pm

7:00 pm

8:00 pm

NACK: Time   **Hours Since Dinner:** Time

te/drank:

EAT!

9:00 pm

0:00 pm

NACK: Time   **Hours Since Snack:** Time

te/drank:

EAT!

1:00 pm

Time I Went to Bed: Time

FOOD LOVERS FAT LOSS SNACK IDEAS

Small Bag of Chips

Slice of Bread with Peanut Butter

1/2 Turkey Sandwich

Cheese & Crackers

Fruit

Nutrition Bar

Leftovers from Lunch or Dinner

NOTES

DAY 2

Yesterday, you started to speed up your metabolism by eating more often.
Today you are going to learn how to use the right combinations
of foods to even out blood sugar levels and switch your body into
Fat Burning Mode everytime you eat.

DAY 2: LEARN TO MAKE A
FAT LOSS PLATE

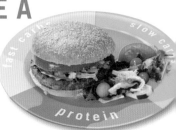

Starting today you are going to make sure one of the meals you eat – either Lunch or Dinner - is a **Food Lovers Fat Loss Meal**. It's remarkably easy to do. Simply read the first 29 pages of the ***How to Make a Fat Loss Plate*** booklet and follow the simple guidelines. In it you'll find the key to this program – the simple secret that will allow you to eat your favorite foods – at every single meal – and reduce your waistline every single week.

How Your Body Processes Food

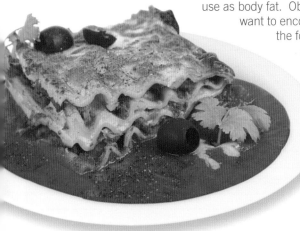

To truly understand the power of the proportions that comprise a **Food Lovers Fat Loss Plate**, it's important to first understand something about how your body processes food. When you eat or drink something your body does one of two things with it: Either it burns it for energy or it stores it for later use as body fat. Obviously, to lose fat and stay lean you want to encourage your body to burn more of the food you eat as energy and discourage it from storing that food as fat. The way you eat your food – the combinations you eat them in – can have a huge effect on how that happens. The way you switch your body from "Fat Storing Mode" to "Fat Burning Mode" is by eating in a way that keeps your blood sugar levels low and even.

MANAGING BLOOD SUGAR LEVELS
The Key to Permanent Fat Loss

The significant factor in whether your body is in Fat Storing Mode or Fat Burning Mode is the amount of sugar in your bloodstream. Sugar in your blood comes from carbohydrates. A carbohydrate, in the most simple terms, is anything that once grew in the ground or is refined from some-thing that once grew in the ground. Obviously, that includes all **fruits** and **vegetables**, but it also includes **sugar**, (which comes from sugar cane, corn syrup, etc.), **breads**, **pastas** (which come from grains) and many **alcoholic beverages** (which are distilled or fermented from grains or sugars).

Every time you eat any carbohydrate, whether it's a baked potato, a piece of chocolate cake or a glass of wine, the first thing your body does is convert it into a sugar called Glucose – which it will then use for energy or, more often, store as fat!

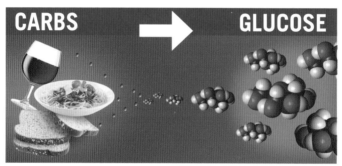

Every **Carb** you eat gets converted into Glucose (a form of sugar) in your body which can trigger the release of "Insulin," the body's primary fat storing hormone.

Why Carbs Have Gotten Such a Bad Rap

If you've read anything about weight loss over the last 10 years you've probably seen one article or another arguing that carbs are the main reason we get fat. The reason that carbs are so often blamed as the cause of weight gain is that when carbs are converted into Glucose in your body they can trigger the release of a hormone called "Insulin." **Insulin is your body's primary fat storing hormone**. It's known as the fat storing hormone because one of its main duties is to get excess sugar out of your bloodstream as quickly as possible (so it doesn't damage your arteries). And that generally means *storing it as fat*. **So... carbs can, indeed, cause you to gain weight... if you eat them in the wrong way.** But, by making some simple changes to the WAY you eat carbs, you can still eat them but do so in a way that keeps your blood sugar, and insulin levels low throughout the day so your body doesn't switch into "Fat Storing Mode."

The Difference Between
FAST CARBS and SLOW CARBS

The important thing to understand about Carbs is: **All Carbs are NOT created equal**. There are actually two different types: **Fast Carbs** and **Slow Carbs**. The primary difference between the two is how quickly they are converted into sugar in your body. The quicker they are converted to glucose the more likely they are to "spike" your insulin levels and switch your body into "Fat Storing Mode." Naturally, **Fast Carbs** convert to sugar quickly while **Slow Carbs** convert much more slowly.

Slow Carbs are foods like fibrous vegetables, greens, beans, berries, etc. They tend to have lots of fiber and other nutrients that slow down their conversion to sugar. **Fast Carbs** are foods like potatoes, rice, sweet fruits and foods high in sugar and processed flour like sweets, bread and pasta. Because they are converted very quickly, sometimes almost instantaneously, into glucose in your body, **Fast Carbs** have the greatest potential to "spike" your insulin levels and switch your body into "Fat Storing Mode." **But Fast Carbs don't have to be bad**. You can still eat them. You just have to learn to eat them in the **right way**.

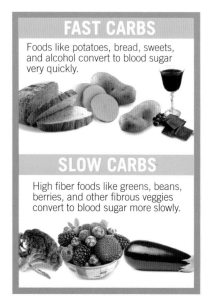

FAST CARBS

Foods like potatoes, bread, sweets, and alcohol convert to blood sugar very quickly.

SLOW CARBS

High fiber foods like greens, beans, berries, and other fibrous veggies convert to blood sugar more slowly.

The Fat Loss Plate –
The Key to Eating *ANYTHING YOU WANT!*

And that's where the Fat Loss Plate comes in. A Fat Loss Plate is the right combination of **Proteins**, **Fast Carbs** and/or **Slow Carbs** in the right proportions to slow down the conversion of carbs to blood sugar and keep insulin levels low. Essentially, these meals switch your body out of "Fat Storing Mode" and put it into "Fat Burning Mode".

And the great news is: you can make a Fat Loss Plate with just about anything! Pasta, bread, lasagna, Mexican food, desserts, even wine and chocolate can all be a part of every meal if you want. The **Food Lovers Fat Loss Plate** allows you to eat all your favorite foods – even the most decadent **Fast Carbs** – in a way that causes your body to lose weight rather than gain weight. And that is the real key to the **Food Lovers Fat Loss System**. Since you aren't depriving yourself of a single one of the foods you love, you can finally stick to an eating plan that will allow you to keep the weight off for the rest of your life.

DO THIS TODAY

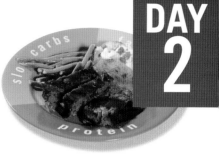

1 **Learn To Make A Fat Loss Plate**
Today, you are going to take your fat loss to the next level by making either your Lunch or Dinner a **Food Lovers Fat Loss Plate**. You'll find all the info you need in the *How to Make a Fat Loss Plate* booklet.

2 **Choose 3 Fat Loss Plates You Love & Write Them Down**
The key to permanent weight loss is to make sure that you love everything you eat. If you enjoy every meal, why would you ever change? Don't let yourself get into a rut where you eat the same thing every day because "it's easy," or "it's the only thing I have in the house." There are literally hundreds of recipes for Fat Loss Plates on the plan. Go through the *Classic Comfort Foods Recipe Cards*, *The Love to Eat Cookbook*, the *Million Meals Menu Planner*, and write down 3 to 6 Fat Loss Meals that you will love to eat on the Lunch (page 62) or Dinner (page 68) sections of the *How to Make a Fat Loss Plate* booklet. Then you'll never have to wonder what's for Lunch or Dinner.

> **Everyday Family Favorite Lunches**
> When I have time to make a proper Lunch, these are
> 1. Sloppy Joes
> 2. Chicken Noodle Soup
> 3. Joe's Homemade Chili
>
> **On The Run**
> Days when I'm in a hurry, I'll eat one of these Foo
> 1. Turkey Sandwich
> 2. Leftover Meatloaf with ve
> 3. Banana Berry Smoothie
>
> **Sunday Afternoon Feasts**
> When it's time to make something truly decad
> these are the Lunches I'll make.
> 1. Turkey & Gravy & Mashed
> 2. Chicken Pot Pie
> 3. Lasagna

3 **Upgrade Your Snacks**
While you continue to ramp up your metabolism by eating every 2 to 3 hours, starting today you are going to accelerate your results by making sure all your snacks meet the simple guidelines of a **Food Lovers Fat Loss Snack**. The opening pages of the *Snack and Treat Guide* will give you all the details you need to know to use great tasting **Food Lovers** snacks to keep your body in "Fat Burning Mode" all day long. And if you really want to accelerate your results, check out the instructions for Accelerator Snacks. They are specially designed for maximum results during your *21 Day Metabolism Makeover*.

4 **Get Ready for Tomorrow**
Starting tomorrow you are going to jump start your metabolism from the moment you wake up with a **Food Lovers Breakfast**. So sometime today, read over the section on **Food Lovers Breakfasts** in the *How to Make a Fat Loss Plate* booklet (pages 54 to 60) and make sure you have the foods you need to make a tasty, fat burning morning meal.

You're On Your Way...
You've now learned the two most important steps that are the basis of the Food Lovers Fat Loss System, a great start to being lean and healthy forever!

DAY 2

LEARN TO MAKE A FAT LOSS PLATE

Follow the instructions in *How to Make a Fat Loss Plate* and make either your Lunch or Dinner a Fat Loss Plate. By combining your foods in the right combinations and right proportions, you will begin to *"Optimize Your Glycemic Profile"* and switch your body from "Fat Storing Mode" to "Fat Burning Mode"

✓ TO DO'S
(check when done)

- [ ] Listen to the **Day 2** Audio Program
- [ ] Make a Fat Loss Plate for Lunch or Dinner
- [ ] Eat every 2 to 3 hours up to 1 hour before bed
- [ ] Choose only **Food Lovers Snacks** today
- [ ] Read Pages 1 to 29 of *How to Make a Fat Loss Plate*
- [ ] Get ready for tomorrow's Breakfast
- [ ] _____
- [ ] _____
- [ ] _____
- [ ] _____

TODAY'S CALLS

_____
_____
_____
_____
_____
_____
_____
_____

TODAY'S SCHEDULE

B-FAST / SNACK: Time   **Mins. Since Waking Up:** Time

I ate/drank:

EAT!

7:00 am

8:00 am

9:00 am

B-FAST / SNACK: Time   **Hours Since Breakfast:** Time

I ate/drank:

EAT!

10:00 am

11:00 am

12:00 pm

LUNCH / SNACK: Time   **Hours Since Snack:** Time

I ate/drank:

EAT!   SLOW CARB / FAST CARB / PROTEIN

1:00 pm

2:00 pm

SNACK: Time   **Hours Since Lunch:** Time

I ate/drank:

EAT!

EXERCISE   ■ YES   ■ NO   TIME [   ]

What/how much?

AT EVERY MEAL, ASK YOURSELF 2 QUESTIONS:

1. What's my Protein?
A Protein is anything that flew, walked or swam (plus soy).

2. What's my Carb?
A Carb is anything that once grew from the ground.

To keep your metabolism running at its fastest, every meal will have a combination of **Protein** plus **Fast Carbs** and/or **Slow Carbs**.

TODAY'S SCHEDULE

3:00 pm

4:00 pm

5:00 pm

DINNER: Time   **Hours Since Snack:** Time

ate/drank:

EAT! Protein
SLOW CARB
FAST CARB
PROTEIN

6:00 pm

7:00 pm

8:00 pm

SNACK: Time   **Hours Since Dinner:** Time

ate/drank:

EAT! Protein

9:00 pm

10:00 pm

SNACK: Time   **Hours Since Snack:** Time

ate/drank:

EAT! Protein

11:00 pm

          Time I Went to Bed: Time

FOOD LOVERS FAT LOSS MEAL COMBINATIONS

VERSION A

1 Portion Each:
Protein, Fast Carb and
Slow Carb

VERSION B

1 Portion Protein and
2 to 3 Portions Slow Carbs

VERSION C

or

1 Portion Protein and
1 Portion Fast Carb

NOTES

You're now eating in a way that keeps your body in **"Fat Burning Mode"** throughout the day. Today we're going to make sure you start burning fat as soon as you wake up.

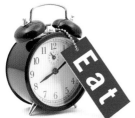

DAY 3:
EAT BREAKFAST
AS SOON AS YOU WAKE UP

Today, you are going to make a Food Lovers Meal for Breakfast and eat it within 60 minutes of waking up. If you can't stomach a big Breakfast as soon as you wake then at least eat a **Food Lovers Snack** and eat your full Breakfast 2 to 3 hours later. But don't wait to eat. Make sure you eat something within one hour, preferably 60 minutes, of waking up.

Why They Call It Break-"FAST"

Breakfast got its name because when you wake up you've actually been fasting for the entire time you've been sleeping, so when you eat after waking up, you are literally "breaking your fast." We already know that when you aren't eating for extended periods of time your metabolism slows down. Eating breakfast within 60 minutes of waking essentially "jump starts" your metabolism. It heats up your body's fat burning furnace so that it can start burning off excess body fat as early as possible. Remember, with **Food Lovers**, frequent eating is how we fire up our metabolism and shed pounds!

IMPORTANT! Please do not be tempted to skip this activity. In many ways, Breakfast really is the most important meal of the day. It not only fires up your metabolism first thing in the morning, but it also gives you a much needed energy boost to start your day.   Even if you're not typically a "Breakfast Person", please realize that eating soon after you awaken is critically important to safe and effective fat loss. You don't have to eat a full meal -- a simple snack will do -- just be sure to eat something. Give it a try for the duration of the *21 Day Metabolism Makeover* and you're sure to experience for yourself a noticeable improvement in how you look and feel. Plus, there are so many delicious choices there's bound to be something you'll enjoy!

Check out **The Love to Eat Cookbook** and the **Classic Comfort Food Recipe Cards** for some of the tastiest Breakfasts you've ever had in your life. You'll find recipes and directions for quick and easy meals like our delicious Mocha Eye Opener Smoothie or a simple bowl of cereal, or fancy feasts like the Tuscan Omelet or Food Lovers Biscuits and Gravy. There's even a recipe for an Egg and Cheese English Muffin that's just as tasty as the one at the fast food place. Find three of your favorites, then jot them down on page 60 of **How to Make a Fat Loss Plate**.

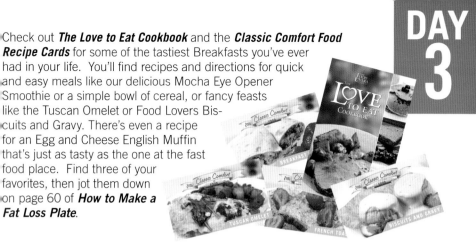

HOW THEY MAKE
SUMO WRESTLERS FAT

There's only one sport where they actually aim to gain as much body fat as possible: Sumo Wrestling. According to their philosophy - here is what a sumo wrestler does to get fat:

1. Skip Breakfast. By depriving their bodies of food after eight hours of sleep (fasting), they never get their metabolism going so they burn less calories during the day.

2. Exercise on an empty stomach. With no food for fuel, their metabolic rate stays low so they burn less calories during their workout.

3. Eat just a couple of meals a day. One famous Sumo wrestler is reported to eat 10 bowls of stew, eight bowls of rice, 130 pieces of sushi, and 25 portions of barbecued beef all in one meal… and still have room for dessert. Their bodies can only process so much food at once, so the rest gets stored as fat.

4. Take a nap after eating. After eating, they sleep for at least four hours - again keeping their metabolism slow.

5. Drink alcohol in excess. It has been reported that Sumo Wrestlers drink upward of 100 bottles of beer at a time which increases Cortisol levels and leads to fat deposits around the abdomen creating their famous "beer bellies" which helps stabilize them in the ring.

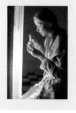

6. Eat late in the day. Going to bed with full stomachs means that their bodies must respond to the huge flood of nutrients with a rush of insulin, forcing their bodies to store the food as fat.

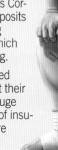

THE MYTH OF WILLPOWER

When people fall off a diet plan they generally blame themselves, thinking they lacked the willpower to skip meals or overcome the cravings. The fact of the matter is when you go four or five hours or more without eating (particularly once your metabolism speeds up) you will become SO hungry that you simply will not be able to control yourself. It has nothing to do with willpower. It's just plain hunger, pure and simple, and no one can resist.

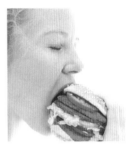

On the **Food Lovers Fat Loss System**, extreme hunger should never be a problem since you are eating all the time. In fact, if you are getting uncomfortably hungry on this program - *you are not eating enough*.

PERCEIVED HUNGER INDEX

Use the following scale to gauge your Hunger Level. If you find yourself at a 2 or 1, eat a snack - even if you've got a meal coming up soon. If you let yourself get too hungry, you're almost guaranteed to overeat. After adding a snack, just wait at least an hour then get right back on schedule.

*Wait at least 20 minutes after eating to gauge your Hunger Level.

*Also, make sure you have been drinking plenty of water. Dehydration often disguises itself as hunger, particularly if you are craving salty, crunchy foods like chips, crackers, etc.

NEVER LET YOURSELF GET TO A 1 OR 0 !

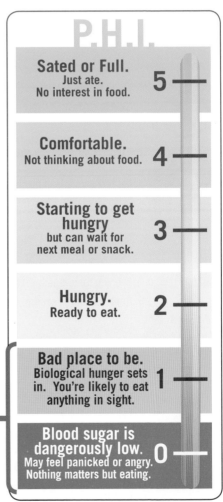

P.H.I.

Sated or Full. Just ate. No interest in food. **5**

Comfortable. Not thinking about food. **4**

Starting to get hungry but can wait for next meal or snack. **3**

Hungry. Ready to eat. **2**

Bad place to be. Biological hunger sets in. You're likely to eat anything in sight. **1**

Blood sugar is dangerously low. May feel panicked or angry. Nothing matters but eating. **0**

Now that you've kick-started your metabolism first thing in the day, here are some tips to keep your metabolism running at its fastest all day long.

- Meal times are calculated from the time you <u>begin</u> eating, not when you <u>finish</u> eating your meal or snack. For example, if you start eating Breakfast at 8:00 a.m., you should start eating your first snack between 10:00 and 11:00 a.m., which is 2 to 3 hours later.

- **If it's time for a meal but you can't get a full meal, then eat a snack.** You can have a full Fat Loss Meal next time it is time to eat. The most important thing is to eat something every 2 to 3 hours.

- **Don't forget dessert** – Your 2 to 3 hour eating schedule continues into the evening all the way up to an hour before you go to bed. So if you eat Dinner at 6:00 and don't go to bed til midnight, you're due for another snack at around 8:00 and another around 10:00 or 10:30.

DO THIS TODAY

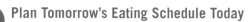

1 Eat Breakfast as Soon as You Get Up

By now your metabolism is racing - you are eating **Food Lovers Fat Loss Snacks** between meals all the way up to one hour before bed (Accelerator Snacks if you really want fast results), and either your Lunch or Dinner is a Fat Loss Plate. Today, you'll make sure you kick-start your fat loss first thing in the morning by eating a **Food Lovers Fat Loss Breakfast** within thirty minutes of waking up.

2 Plan Tomorrow's Eating Schedule Today

Since eating regularly is so very important to long term success on this program, you're going to make sure you're eating schedule is perfect tomorrow. So tonight, fill in your eating schedule for tomorrow. Decide now what time you are going to wake up and enter your eating times in your Planner Pages making sure there is never more than 3 hours between meals. Go through the recipes in the program and choose the meals you'll be preparing and the snacks you'll be eating tomorrow. Then fill these meals and snacks in on your Planner Page for tomorrow and make sure you have the food you're planning to eat on hand so there is no way you can fail.

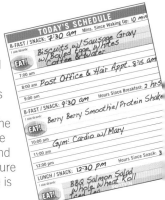

3 Get Ready for Tomorrow

Starting tomorrow you are going to upgrade your third and final meal to a **Food Lovers Fat Loss Plate**. To make sure you are ready, go through the cookbook and recipe cards today, choose your favorites and make sure you've got the food you need on hand to make three Fat Loss Plates tomorrow (breakfast, lunch and dinner) so you can keep your body's fat burning engine running on high all day long. And remember you can make a Fat Loss Plate at all your favorite restaurants as well. Just read the ***Eating Out Advisor*** booklet before you go.

DAY 3

EAT BREAKFAST
WITHIN 60 MINUTES OF WAKING UP

Within an hour of waking up, eat a **Food Lovers Fat Loss Breakfast** to switch your Body into "Fat Burning Mode" as soon as you start your day.

✓ TO DO'S
(check when done)

- [ ] Listen to the **Day 3** Audio Program
- [ ] Eat a Fat Loss Breakfast within 60 minutes of waking
- [ ] Eat a Fat Loss Lunch OR Dinner
- [ ] Fill out eating schedule for tomorrow
- [ ] Get ready to make 3 Fat Loss Meals tomorrow
- [ ] _____
- [ ] _____
- [ ] _____
- [ ] _____
- [ ] _____

TODAY'S CALLS

_____
_____
_____
_____
_____
_____
_____
_____
_____

TODAY'S SCHEDULE

B-FAST / SNACK: Time   **Mins. Since Waking Up:** Time

I ate/drank:

EAT! Protein   SLOW CARB
                    FAST CARB
                    PROTEIN

7:00 am

8:00 am

9:00 am

B-FAST / SNACK: Time   **Hours Since Breakfast:** Time

I ate/drank:

EAT! Protein

10:00 am

11:00 am

12:00 pm

LUNCH / SNACK: Time   **Hours Since Snack:** Time

I ate/drank:

EAT! Protein   SLOW CARB
                    FAST CARB
                    PROTEIN

1:00 pm

2:00 pm

SNACK: Time   **Hours Since Lunch:** Time

I ate/drank:

EAT! Protein

EXERCISE   ☐ YES   ☐ NO   TIME [   ]

What/how much?
_____
_____

By skipping breakfast, the metabolic rate may drop 4% to 5% below normal which can result in a weight gain of 1 pound every seven weeks, even if calorie intake stays the same.

TODAY'S SCHEDULE

:00 pm

:00 pm

:00 pm

NNER:	Time	Hours Since Snack:	Time
e/drank:			

AT!

SLOW CARB
FAST CARB
PROTEIN

:00 pm

:00 pm

00 pm

ACK:	Time	Hours Since Dinner:	Time
e/drank:			

AT!

:00 pm

:00 pm

ACK:	Time	Hours Since Snack:	Time
e/drank:			

AT!

:00 pm

Time I Went to Bed: Time

OTES

FOOD LOVERS
QUICK BREAKFAST
IDEAS

Bowl of Cereal
Pg 58 in BREAKFAST section
of *How to Make a Fat Loss Plate*

French Toast
Classic Comfort Food
Recipe Card

Food Lovers Fat Loss Muffin
Classic Comfort Food
Recipe Card

Egg Sandwich
Pg 46 in BREAKFAST section
of *The Love to Eat Cookbook*

Family Favorite Pancakes
Classic Comfort Food
Recipe Card

Unlike many diet plans that ask you to cut out breads and sweets, today you'll learn how to make simple changes that make it possible for you to continue eating them in a way that will cause your body to lose weight rather than gain weight.

DAY 4:
EAT MORE
HEALTHY BREADS AND SWEETS

During the first 21 days of the program while we are trying to reset your metabolism and get it burning fat as fast as possible, we are going to focus on the foods that really accelerate fat burning and avoid those that have the greatest potential to slow things down. To do that, you are going to become a Label Detective and learn how to spot those ingredients which are most likely to switch your body from "Fat Burning Mode" to "Fat Storing Mode." **Then, for the next 17 days you'll ramp up your metabolism by avoiding breads and sweets that have Refined Sugars listed among the first three ingredients on the nutrition label, and choosing breads with at least 3g of Fiber per serving.**

The Biggest "Enemies of Fat Loss"

On Day 2 you learned how **Fast Carbs** can cause your insulin levels to rise which can throw your body into "Fat Storing Mode." Today, we're going to learn a bit more about **Fast Carbs**. Just as all carbs are NOT created equal, neither are all **Fast Carbs** created equal – some are faster than others. And the faster they are, the more likely they are to compromise your blood sugar levels.

SUPER Fast Carbs –
the Worst of the Worse

When you pull an ear of corn off a stalk or a bunch of wheat from the field, it is loaded with fiber and other nutrients which slow the rate that the corn or wheat is converted into sugar in your body. But when that corn gets processed into corn syrup and used to sweeten your soda pop, or when that wheat gets ground and bleached into white flour, all the fiber and other nutrients get stripped away. We are left with a **Fast Carb** in, essentially, its purest form – with nothing to slow down its conversion to sugar in your blood stream. As a general rule, **the more "processed" and "refined" a carbohydrate is the greater its potential for "spiking" your insulin level and throwing your body into "Fat Storing Mode."** And unfortunately, so much of the food we eat today is loaded with two of the most refined carbohydrates – sugar and white flour.

Simple Sugar
Straight from Your Table to Your Blood Stream

Most of the sugar we eat – whether it's in candy, soda, baked goods or straight from the sugar bowl into our coffee or onto our cereal – started out in this world as a "whole" or unrefined food. In most cases, it began as either a tall, fibrous grass called Sugar Cane or as good ol' Corn. Then, in the refining process, these plants are stripped of all the "food" portion – all the fiber and many of the nutrients – and what is left is just the sugar.

If you remember, the biggest key to whether a food will cause your body to go into "Fat Storing Mode" is how quickly it is converted to sugar in your body. Well, in the case of these simple sugars and sweeteners the manufacturers have already done most of the work your body would normally do. They've already converted these plants into sugar which means they can be converted to blood sugar so quickly that (if we don't slow the conversion process somehow as we do with a **Fat Loss Plate**) they are almost guaranteed to "spike" your insulin levels and throw your body into "Fat Storing Mode."

Refined Sugars

1. Sugar
2. High Fructose Corn Syrup
3. Brown Sugar
4. Dextrose
5. Maltose
6. Corn Syrup
7. Malt Syrup
8. Maple Syrup

Since these sugars have such potential to compromise your blood sugar level, we're going to try to minimize them as much as possible during your *21 Day Metabolism Makeover.* Unfortunately, that can be a bit tricky because these refined sugars hide behind so many different names. Look for the following names on your food labels and avoid foods that have any of them listed as one of the first 3 ingredients.

HOW TO READ A NUTRITION LABEL

Nutrition labels list ingredients in order by amount. So a product that lists "high fructose corn syrup" as the first ingredient has more high fructose corn syrup in it than anything else. Many products have multiple types of these "processed" and "simple" sugars and grains in one product. The more they have, the more Refined Sugar is in the product. Also, watch out for the use of parentheses. You are looking for the first 3 ingredients NOT in parentheses.

But, Wait, I Want My Sweets...

Slow down! We're not asking you to give up sweets (and any weight loss plan that does is doomed to failure). We're just asking you to focus on sweeteners that don't have such a negative effect on your blood sugar level for the next 17 days. Look for products sweetened with low or no calorie alternatives like **Splenda**, **Stevia** or **Neotame**. There are also a wide variety of more natural, less processed alternatives that are delicious, healthier substitutes for all your favorite recipes like **evaporated cane juice, whole fruit and fruit juices, raw or organic agave nectar, xylitol, brown rice syrup and Sucanat**. You'll find a detailed list of less processed or no calorie alternatives on page 3 of *The Love to Eat Cookbook*. With so many choices, you really can have your cake and eat it too.

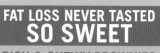

FAT LOSS NEVER TASTED
SO SWEET

RICH & CHEWY BROWNIES

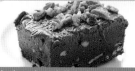

This decadent delight is made with only fat burning ingredients.

Ingredients:
Dry
- 1 cup Evaporated Cane Juice
- 1 cup 100% whole wheat flour (use rice flour if gluten-sensitive)
- 1/2 cup natural unsweetened cocoa powder
- 1 heaping scoop of vanilla protein powder
- 1 tsp baking soda
- 2 TBSP 60% cocoa semi-sweet chocolate chips
- 1/2 cup walnut pieces

Wet
- 2 egg whites
- 1 cup unsweetened applesauce
- 2 TBSP original soy milk (we recommend Silk®)
- 1 tsp vanilla extract

Method:
Preheat oven to 350 degrees. Set aside 1 TBSP of both the chocolate chips and the walnuts for the topping, then mix remaining dry ingredients together in a big bowl. It is best if you get the lumps out of each dry ingredient before you add it to the bowl. In a separate bowl, mix wet ingredients together. Then, slowly add the dry ingredients to the wet, mixing well to prevent lumps from forming. Spray an 8x8 baking pan with cooking spray. Pour the brownie mixture into the pan. Top with the leftover walnut pieces and chocolate chips. Bake for 30-40 minutes. Cool and serve. Makes 16 Servings.

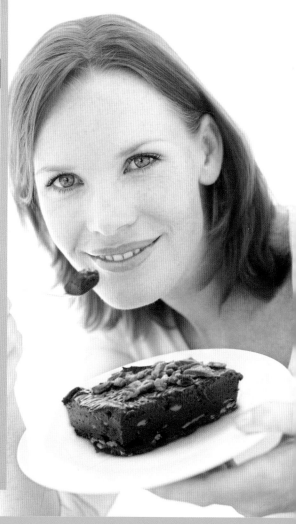

DAY 4

Breads & Flour

Like sugar, processed grains in the form of flours can be high in calories, low in nutrition and responsible for triggering a rush of insulin which can slow or even halt weight loss. They'll be listed on nutrition labels as **bleached, enriched** or **white flour**. Conversely, foods such as bread made with 100% whole wheat flour and cereals made with whole grains are healthy, high in fiber, and aid in weight loss as well as the prevention of many diseases.

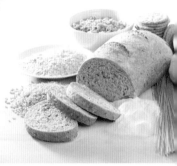

How To Choose Breads and Rolls

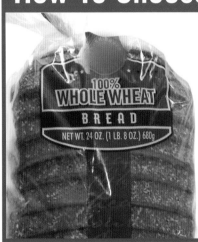

The simplest way to choose breads and rolls that won't quickly send you into "Fat Storing Mode" is to follow these two guidelines:

1 **Avoid any Refined Sugar in the first 3 ingredients**

2 **Choose breads that have at least 3g of fiber per serving**

By following these two simple guidelines, you'll automatically avoid those products that are made primarily of processed grains.

What to Expect

By choosing foods and beverages that aren't loaded with Refined Sugars have at least 3g of fiber, you are naturally eating what we refer to as "nutrient dense" foods which will have a tremendous, positive effect on your metabolism. The fiber and nutrients slow the conversion of these carbs to sugar in your blood – which prevents a large release of insulin and keeps your body in "Fat Burning Mode."

But you will notice other benefits as well. By eating unprocessed foods and foods higher in fiber, you're going to experience an increase in overall mood, energy and you are less likely to feel bloated. The best part is that it's become easy to find these healthier alternatives throughout the country, and you'll never feel like you're missing anything.

DO THIS TODAY

1 **Eat More Healthy Breads & Sweets**
Starting today and for the rest of your *21 Day Metabolism Makeover*, you are going to begin to optimize your metabolism **by choosing foods and beverages that do NOT have Refined Sugars listed in the first three ingredients on the nutritional label. Also choose breads that have at least 3g of fiber per serving.** If you have trouble finding brands that meet this criteria, you may choose to focus on potatoes, rice and other "whole food" **Fast Carbs** for the first 21 days.

2 **Make All 3 Meals Fat Loss Plates**
Starting today, upgrade your third and final meal to a **Food Lovers Fat Loss Plate**. That means for the next 17 days, you will be eating Fat Loss Plates for all three of your meals and snacking in between meals every 2 to 3 hours all the way up to one hour before bed to keep your body in "Fat Burning Mode" all day long.

3 **Upgrade Your Pantry**
It's harder to eat healthy when you are constantly faced with the marketing on the labels of foods that are loaded with Refined Sugars. So go through your pantry, read the labels, look for these "Enemies of Fat Loss" and for the rest of your *21 Day Metabolism Makeover*, get them out of your sight. Donate them to a shelter, give them to a friend or just tuck them away. Then head out to the store and stock up on healthier choices. Get some whole grain flour and healthier sweeteners, then go through the *Snack and Treat Guide* and make a list of snacks and treats that you'll truly enjoy and fill up your pantry. Make sure you have "Accelerator Snacks" available, as they're guaranteed to maximize weight loss during the first 21 days. **Try to find a substitute that you like just as well for every food you discard today**.

DAY 4

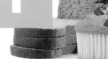

EAT MORE
HEALTHY BREADS & SWEETS

For the next 17 days, maximize your metabolism by choosing only prepackaged foods and beverages that do <u>NOT</u> contain refined sugars in the <u>first three</u> ingredients of the nutrition label, and bread with at least <u>3 grams</u> of fiber per serving.

✓ TO DO'S
(check when done)

- ☐ Listen to the **Day 4** Audio Program
- ☐ Choose only healthy breads and sweets
- ☐ Eat a Fat Loss Plate for every meal
- ☐ Eat every 2 to 3 hours up to 1 hour before bed
- ☐ Get the "Enemies of Fat Loss" out of your pantry
- ☐ Stock up on Accelerator Snacks
- ☐ _____
- ☐ _____
- ☐ _____
- ☐ _____
- ☐ _____

TODAY'S CALLS

_____
_____
_____
_____
_____
_____
_____
_____

TODAY'S SCHEDULE

B-FAST / SNACK: Time   **Mins. Since Waking Up:** Time

I ate/drank:

EAT!   SLOW CARB
           FAST CARB
           PROTEIN

7:00 am

8:00 am

9:00 am

B-FAST / SNACK: Time   **Hours Since Breakfast:** Time

I ate/drank:

EAT!

10:00 am

11:00 am

12:00 pm

LUNCH / SNACK: Time   **Hours Since Snack:** Time

I ate/drank:

EAT!   SLOW CARB
           FAST CARB
           PROTEIN

1:00 pm

2:00 pm

SNACK: Time   **Hours Since Lunch:** Time

I ate/drank:

EAT!

EXERCISE   ☐ YES   ☐ NO   TIME _____

What/how much?
_____
_____

GRAIN FOR GRAIN - A BETTER CHOICE

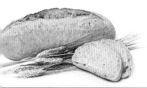

Eating more whole grains has been shown to reduce the risk of heart disease, cancer and diabetes, plus recent studies suggest that whole grains may also lower triglycerides (cholesterol), improve insulin control and slow the buildup of arterial plaque. Oh, the power of the whole grain!

TODAY'S SCHEDULE

3:00 pm

4:00 pm

5:00 pm

DINNER: Time   **Hours Since Snack:** Time

ate/drank:

EAT!   SLOW CARB
FAST CARB
PROTEIN

6:00 pm

7:00 pm

8:00 pm

SNACK: Time   **Hours Since Dinner:** Time

ate/drank:

EAT!

9:00 pm

10:00 pm

SNACK: Time   **Hours Since Snack:** Time

ate/drank:

EAT!

11:00 pm

Time I Went to Bed: Time

NOTES

OUR FAVORITE FAT LOSS BAKED GOODS

Our Favorite Breads
1. Trader Joe's® 7 Grain Sourdough Whole Wheat Mini-Loaf
2. Milton's® 100% Whole Wheat
3. Vogel's® 12 Grain Toast

Our Favorite Cereals
1. Nature's Path® Blueberry Cinnamon
2. Trader Joe's® Raisin Bran Clusters
3. O Organics® Multi Circles Organic Multigrain

Our Favorite Snacks
1. Kettle® Brand Baked Potato Chips
2. Frito-Lay Baked Tostitos Scoops® Tortilla Chips
3. Frito-Lay® Sunchips Original Flavor Multigrain Snacks

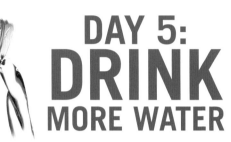

Congratulations on arriving at Day 5!
You've already learned how to use food to speed up your metabolism.
Today you are going to do the same thing with water.

DAY 5:
DRINK
MORE WATER

Imagine speeding up your metabolism by adding just one 8 oz. glass of water to your day. Better yet, how about releasing 5 pounds of fat in 1 month by simply drinking more water? Just as eating every 2 to 3 hours is a proven method for speeding up your metabolism, so is drinking water throughout the day. An increase in water consumption alone can aid in releasing up to 3 to 5 pounds over the next 16 days of your *21 Day Metabolism Makeover*. **So start drinking at least one extra glass of water today. The goal is to eventually work your way up to a minimum of 12 (8 oz.) glasses a day to maximize fat metabolism. But for today, just start drinking MORE**.

Make it your goal to drink water as often as possible: before, during and after meals and snacks.

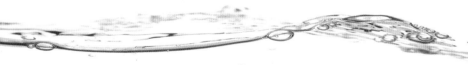

The Magic of Water

It may seem unbelievable, but one of the simplest ways to increase weight loss and improve overall health is to drink more water. In fact, it may be one of the single most important factors in releasing fat.

Your body requires adequate hydration to function properly. Without it, you may experience a host of unpleasant symptoms including: increased hunger and cravings, headaches, fatigue, fluid retention, bloating and... weight gain. On the other hand, increasing water consumption will help:
- Naturally suppress appetite
- Prevent water retention and bloating (swollen feet, legs, hands and belly)
- Help your muscle tissue work more efficiently to burn more calories all day long
- Rid the body of toxins
- Prevent and relieve constipation
- Increase the efficiency of your metabolism and help your body burn fat

Why Water Is
The Key to Fat Metabolism…

It's no secret that water is a key ingredient for maximum fat loss. Keeping your body hydrated helps accelerate your metabolism and means you're burning more fat! In fact, studies have shown that drinking too little water can cause fat deposits to increase, while drinking more can actually reduce fat deposits. It all has to do with how your body processes fat.

It starts with the kidneys. They need adequate water to work well. If they don't get it, they dump some of their workload onto the liver. That's where the trouble begins because the liver is one of the key organs involved in metabolizing stored fat into energy. When the kidneys aren't working to capacity, the liver has to pick up the slack. And when the liver is doing the work the kidneys should be doing, it can't be doing its job of getting rid of stored fat and turning it into energy to the best of its ability. That means it metabolizes less fat into energy and more fat remains stored in your body. The simple fix: drink more water.

How Can I Add More
Water to My Day?

There are lots of ways to get more water in your day. Beverages like coffee, iced tea, diet soda and other calorie-free beverages count toward your 12 glasses a day. But nothing is as good as plain pure water, so try these tips for **Getting More Water into Your Day:**

❶ Drink one 8 oz. glass of water every hour while at work. By the end of an eight hour day, you will be well on your way. Add two before work and two more in the evening and you're done.

❷ When you have a craving… for anything, drink a glass of water before you do anything else. That craving may be the result of dehydration and the water will help you feel full.

❸ Drink through a straw; you'll tend to take larger sips.

❹ If you are having some fruit juice, cut it one for one with water (50% water / 50% juice).

❺ After each trip to the rest room, drink a glass of water to replenish your system.

❻ If you drink Diet Soda during the day, drink two glasses of water between each 12 oz. soda.

❼ At each meal, drink at least two glasses of water. With each snack, drink one.

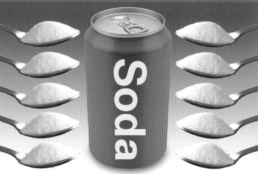

HOW TO STOP FAT LOSS IN ITS TRACKS

12 oz. can = 10 tsp of granulated sugar

When people think about losing weight by "dieting" or "cutting back" they often think exclusively about the food they eat. **The fact is what you drink can often have an even bigger effect on weight loss**. Consider this: one can of regular soda has the equivalent of 10 teaspoons of granulated sugar. And fruit juices are often so loaded with sugar that the American Academy of Pediatrics recommends that infants should not be given <u>ANY</u> fruit juice and that consumption should be severely limited in children. Since soda as well as fruit juice, "energy" drinks and "sports" drinks are essentially nothing but sugar and water, one can or bottle consumed by itself is going to raise insulin levels almost immediately. This is one of the fastest and surest ways to throw yourself into "Fat Storing Mode".

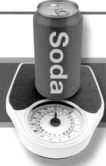

A single can of regular soda per day can make you **gain 15 pounds of body weight per year!**

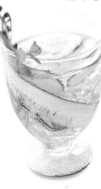

What About Everything Else I Drink?

There truly is no substitute for clean, fresh water! Virtually everything else we drink can contain an ingredient that will slow down or even halt weight loss.

- **Sugar** can "spike" insulin and slow down your metabolism.
- **Sodium (salt)** makes the body retain water, thus increasing weight and bloating.
- **Alcohol** is converted into sugar by the body.
- **Milk (dairy)** can be very high in fat, sugar, and calories.

FOR VARIETY...
These beverages can be substituted occasionally throughout the day.

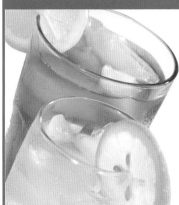

- Coffee
- Iced Tea
- Herb Tea
- Flavored Diet Iced Teas
- Mineral Water
- Diet Sodas
- Club Soda (w/Lemon or Lime)
- Sugar Free Lemonades
- Sparkling Water (Perrier, Pellegrino, etc.)

*We suggest choosing beverages sweetened with Splenda® rather than Aspartame when possible.

How to Drink Yourself Fat

A Venti-sized Java Chip Frappuccino Blended Coffee from Starbucks® has *more* calories **than a Big Mac®** and nearly just as much **fat!!**

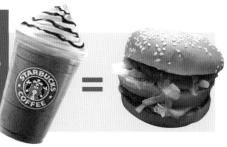

ALCOHOL & WEIGHT LOSS

When you drink alcohol, the liver prioritizes the removal of alcohol from the blood over its other metabolic processes. On average, the liver can detoxify about one ounce of alcohol (which is equal to one mixed drink, one 12-ounce beer, or one 5-ounce glass of wine) in an hour while still maintaining its normal processes, one of which is metabolizing fat. The problem comes when you drink more alcohol than your liver can process while still keeping up with its regular duties (either by drinking in larger quantities or at a faster rate, which many people often do). In addition to its normal chores of filtering your blood and metabolizing fat, your liver will now have to work primarily on the removal of alcohol which means it stops metabolizing fat. Which all boils down to this: **when you drink alcohol, you are more likely to gain fat**.

Furthermore, **alcohol has been found to stimulate the appetite**. As a matter of fact, some doctors have actually prescribed one alcoholic beverage before meals to adults with poor appetites. Lastly, when you drink alcohol, you are more likely to increase your consumption of daily calories. When you're interested in releasing fat, it is important that you consume fewer calories than required for your body to stay at your current weight. When you choose to drink calories instead of eating them, *you may not feel satisfied and this may induce cravings*. For all these reasons, we suggest that for the next 16 days, in order to revive your slow metabolism and get you burning fat as fast as possible, you avoid alcoholic beverages.

The good news is, once your *21 Day Metabolism Makeover* is over and your metabolism is fully optimized, the *Food Lovers for Life* program will show you how to put alcohol back into your eating plan without slowing your weight loss.

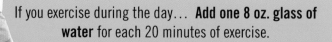

If you exercise during the day... **Add one 8 oz. glass of water** for each 20 minutes of exercise.

DO THIS TODAY

1 **Drink More Water**

Today, you make one of the easiest and most effective tweaks to increase fat loss by simply starting to drink more water. Make sure you drink at least one more glass than you normally do – but remember, in many ways, the more you drink, the more you lose. Try to work your way up to 12 (8 oz.) glasses a day. And, remember for the rest of your *21 Day Metabolism Makeover* you're avoiding refined sugars and flour so make sure you watch out for them in your beverages too.

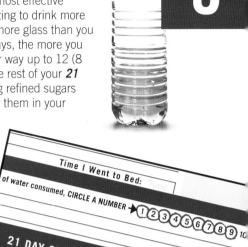

2 **Begin Journaling Your Water Consumption**

Since drinking adequate water is so important to weight loss, starting today you are going to keep track of how many glasses of water you drink. On the lower right portion of your Planner Pages you'll find a series of numbers. Circle one each time you drink an 8 oz. glass of water. Also use your Label Detective skills when enjoying store-bought drinks! Watch out for drinks that are loaded with sugar or fat. Make sure you are keeping track of **everything** you drink, as well as what you eat, in your Planner Pages, so you can learn what beverages have the most effect on your weight.

3 **For the Next 16 Days, Avoid Alcohol**

Since alcohol can slow your weight loss progress - as well as increase cravings - during this induction phase, do the best you can to avoid alcoholic beverages. Once your *21 Day Metabolism Makeover* is done, the *Food Lovers for Life* program will show you how to put wine, beer or even hard liquor back into your eating schedule – every day if you like. It can actually be part of a meal or snack as a **Fast Carb**.

4 **Keep Away from the Scale**

Even though you may be feeling leaner and your clothes are loosening, avoid stepping on the scale until Day 21. Remember, your total body weight can fluctuate 1 to 4 lbs. daily. We've seen cases where weight fluctuates over 10 lbs. just because of water. So be patient...it'll be a nice surprise to see all the weight you've lost at the end of the 21 days!

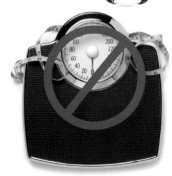

DAY 5

DRINK MORE WATER

Start drinking <u>at least</u> one extra glass of water today – try to work your way up to a minimum of 12 (8 oz) glasses a day to maximize fat metabolism.

✓ TO DO'S
(check when done)

- ☐ Listen to the **Day 5** Audio Program
- ☐ Drink more water
- ☐ Choose only non-alcoholic beverages
- ☐ Eat Breakfast as soon as I get up
- ☐ Eat Food Lovers Fat Loss Snacks and Meals every 2 to 3 hours
- ☐ Choose only healthy breads and sweets
- ☐ _____
- ☐ _____
- ☐ _____
- ☐ _____

TODAY'S CALLS

_____
_____
_____
_____
_____
_____
_____
_____
_____

TODAY'S SCHEDULE

B-FAST / SNACK: Time   **Mins. Since Waking Up:** Time
I ate/drank:

 EAT! Protein

7:00 am

8:00 am

9:00 am

B-FAST / SNACK: Time   **Hours Since Breakfast:** Time
I ate/drank:

EAT! Protein

10:00 am

11:00 am

12:00 pm

LUNCH / SNACK: Time   **Hours Since Snack:** Time
I ate/drank:

EAT! Protein

1:00 pm

2:00 pm

SNACK: Time   **Hours Since Lunch:** Time
I ate/drank:

EAT! Protein

EXERCISE ☐ YES ☐ NO   TIME _____
What/how much?
_____
_____

DAY 5

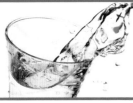
TODAY'S SCHEDULE

3:00 pm

4:00 pm

5:00 pm

DINNER: Time   **Hours Since Snack:** Time

I ate/drank:

EAT!

6:00 pm

7:00 pm

8:00 pm

SNACK: Time   **Hours Since Dinner:** Time

I ate/drank:

EAT!

9:00 pm

10:00 pm

SNACK: Time   **Hours Since Snack:** Time

I ate/drank:

EAT!

11:00 pm

Time I Went to Bed: Time

OUR FAVORITE NO CALORIE BEVERAGES

We tasted the leading brands and these are our favorites.

Diet Coke w/Lime

Sierra Mist Free

Diet Snapple Iced Tea

Boylan's Diet Root Beer

Tropicana Sugar Free Orangeade

Diet Dr. Pepper Berries & Cream

Diet A&W Root Beer

Coke Vanilla Zero

NOTES

1 For each 8 oz. glass of water consumed, **CIRCLE A NUMBER** → 1 2 3 4 5 6 7 8 9 10 11 12

DAY 6

Today we are going to make the last changes to the way you eat, which will make sure your **METABOLISM IS RUNNING ABSOLUTELY AS FAST AS POSSIBLE** for the last two weeks of your *21 Day Metabolism Makeover.*

DAY 6:
EAT MORE
HEALTHY FAT

Many people have grown up thinking that if you eat fat you're going to gain fat. Well, this is not necessarily true. The fact is: your body NEEDS fat to function properly. But just like so many other things, ALL fat is not created equal: some fats are good, some are bad and some are downright ugly. So for the next 15 days we're going to avoid the bad and the ugly and concentrate on the good – which are really good. To do this, you're going to **eat MORE foods high in Mono and Poly Unsaturated Fats** (fish, nuts, healthy oils, etc), **REDUCE foods high in Saturated Fat** (pork, red meat, and dairy products) and **AVOID foods that contain Trans Fats including fried and breaded foods**.

Fat and Fat Loss

Your body needs fat to survive. Good Fats, which are known as **mono-unsaturated** or **poly-unsaturated fats**, are essential for healthy hair, skin and joints, for lowering the risk of heart disease and for many other critical processes in your body. Additionally, fat gives you a feeling of fullness and keeps you from getting hungry too soon. Because these healthy fats are so critical to your health, they are called **"essential" fatty acids**. You'll find them in fish, leafy green vegetables and soy as well as flaxseed, hemp oil, and walnuts to name just a few. You want to concentrate on these healthy fats. Eventually you'll want to get between 30 to 50 grams of healthy fat per day.

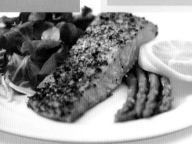

NUTRITION FACTS

1g Protein = 4 calories
1g Carbohydrate = 4 calories
1g Fat = 9 Calories

Unfortunately, not all fats are equally healthful. In fact, some are downright dangerous. And it is critical to know the difference. Additionally, eating too much fat, of any kind, can create challenges when it comes to weight loss because fat is very calorically dense - one gram of fat has more than twice the calories of a gram of **Protein** or **Carbohydrate**. Eating just small amounts of food that are high in fat can add a huge amount of calories to your daily intake. For example, 1 tablespoon of salad dressing can have more than 100 calories - more than the entire salad itself! A glob of butter on your baked potato *can have more calories than the whole potato!*

And that means, even though you are now eating in a way that speeds up your metabolism, if you eat a lot of high fat foods, you're liable to consume so many calories that, no matter how fast your metabolism is working, your body will never be able to convert all the calories into energy and will have to resort to storing the excess as fat.

FAT AND THE FAT LOSS PLATE

Fat is not one of the mandatory ingredients of a Fat Loss Plate because you will get all the Fat your body needs from your protein and carbohydrate sources. Since Fat has so many calories and can slow your metabolism, we encourage you to think of added Fats (dressings, cheese, buttery sauces, the oil you cook with, etc.) as condiments which add flavor to your food rather than being a main ingredient smothering your Fat Loss Plates. Limit Fat to one portion per Fat Loss Plate – a Fatty Protein, a Fatty Fast Carb, or a single serving of Fat.

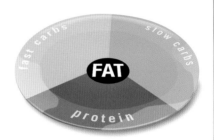

● = **Fat**
Try to limit your intake of added fat per meal to: 1 TBSP - mayonnaise, oil and high-fat dressing and sauces or 1 oz cheese

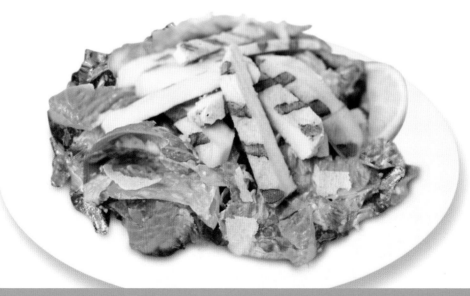

DAY 6

THE BAD FATS
Saturated Fats

Saturated Fats are found in animal products such as steak, butter, and cheese. Saturated Fats have been linked to several health conditions such as hypertension, heart disease, strokes, various forms of cancer and, of course, obesity. All animal sources of **Protein** contain saturated fat. However, turkey breast, chicken breast, and buffalo have far less saturated fat than beef, pork, lamb or duck.

For the next 15 days we want you to choose to avoid **Protein** sources that are high in Saturated Fats. So, when making sausage gravy for instance, use turkey sausage. When eating steak or pork, choose leaner versions and be sure to trim the fat. With chicken, simply remove the skin and you will significantly reduce the amount of Saturated Fats in that meal.

Frying foods adds a significant amount of Saturated and Trans Fats to the serving. On **Food Lovers** we encourage you to roast, grill, sauté, boil, broil or bake your meats.

SATURATED FATS
IN FOOD
Try to keep your daily intake of saturated fats to 10 grams or less.

Food Item (uncooked – per 4 oz serving)	Total Fat (grams)	Saturated Fat (grams)
Bacon - Raw	51.2 g	17.0 g
Pork Sausage, Raw	30.1 g	10.0 g
Prime Rib (Slow Roasted)	25.2 g	10.4 g
Chicken Thigh (Raw with Skin)	17.3 g	5.0 g
T-Bone Steak (Lean, Fat Trimmed, Raw)	16.3 g	6.3 g
Filet Mignon (Lean, Fat Trimmed, Raw)	10.1 g	4.0 g
Turkey Thigh (Raw with Skin)	6.0 g	2.0 g
Salmon (Sockeye, Raw)	9.7 g	1.7 g
Top Sirloin Steak (Lean, Fat Trimmed, Raw)	4.6 g	1.7 g
Fish (Tilapia, Raw)	1.7 g	0.6 g
Chicken Breasts (Raw, Skinless, Meat Only)	1.4 g	0.4 g
Turkey Breasts (Raw, Skinless/Meat Only)	1.5 g	0 g

Trans Fats

Used primarily as a binding agent and to extend the shelf life of many packaged products, **Trans Fats** are fats which were originally healthy, but have gone through a "hydrogenation" process altering their chemical structure and making them extremely unhealthy. In short, **Trans Fats are consider by most experts (including major universities and the World Health Organization) to be the worst thing to happen to our food supply**.

Like sugar, Trans Fats hide behind a variety of names. To ensure that a food does not contain Trans Fatty Acids, regardless of whether the label says "trans fat free" or "no trans fats," look for any of these ingredients listed on the label. ➡

Trans Fats are found in a host of foods including many snack foods, packaged sweets, margarine and many more. Aside from the scientifically proven data that Trans Fats are detrimental to your health, they are also very detrimental to fat loss. **When it comes to Trans Fats, we encourage you to avoid them at all costs**.

DANGER

TRANS FATS

Hydrogenated oils
Partially hydrogenated oils
Fractionated oils
Vegetable shortening
Lard

Deep-Fried and Breaded Foods

If it's fried or breaded, it's likely that it's high in calories and contains Trans Fatty Acids, which are linked to fat gain and health hardships such as type 2 diabetes, hypertension and heart disease so whenever possible, you should look for a more healthful alternative. This is particularly important when eating out. While many restaurants may advertise that their French fries are cooked in oils without Trans Fats such as peanut or extra virgin olive oil, once those oils get heated to the point that they are smoking – as they do in the fryer – *they are converted into Trans Fat by the high temperatures!* So it is very hard to get deep-fried foods at restaurants without Trans Fats. Similarly, when you cook at home over high temperatures, you will want to **choose grape seed oil, safflower oil, avocado oil and macadamia oil** because they have a higher smoking temperature.

During your *21 Day Metabolism Makeover*, instead of eating foods that are fried and breaded (unless you study the label and are sure it is breaded with whole grains and contains NO Trans Fat), choose to bake, boil, broil, grill, steam or stir-fry your food. You'll find recipes for non-fried versions of French fries, fried chicken and all you favorite fried foods in *The Love to Eat Cookbook* and the *Classic Comfort Foods Recipe Cards*.

ZERO TRANS FAT DOESN'T ALWAYS MEAN ZERO TRANS FAT

Nutrition Facts
Serving Size 2 cookies (28g)
Servings Per Container about 7

Amount Per Serving

Calories 140   Calories from Fat 60

% Daily Value*

Total Fat 7g	11 %
Saturated Fat 6g	29 %
Trans Fat 0g	

Ingredients: Sugar, enriched flour (wheat flour, niacin, reduced iron, thiamine mononitrate, riboflavin, folic acid), vegetable shortening (contains one or more of the following partially hydrogenated oils: palm kernel, coconut, soybean, palm), corn syrup, coconut, sweetened condensed milk (milk, sugar), high fruc-

Because information on nutrition labels is based on the percentage of an ingredient in a "serving," it is possible for manufacturers to advertise products as having **NO** Trans Fats even when they do. To be sure, you **MUST** read the ingredient label and look for hydrogenated and fractionated oils.

Choose Healthier Fats

The easiest way to eat more healthy fat is simply to replace unhealthy fats with healthy fat substitutions. For instance, if you enjoy butter on your pancakes, try Earth Balance® or Smart Balance® brands of butter in its place. When making a stir-fry use grape seed oil instead of Crisco®. Avocados are primarily made up of healthy fat and make a great alternative to mayo for your sandwich and it makes a great dip (guacamole).

In the "Fat and the Fat Loss Plate" section of the ***How to Make a Fat Loss Plate*** you'll find a list of recommended healthy fat-based condiments and substitutions.

EXAMPLES OF HEALTHY FAT SOURCES:

- **Ground Flaxseeds**
- **Nuts (i.e., almonds, walnuts)**
- **Oils (i.e., olive, macadamia, coconut, grape seed)**
- **Herbal Supplements (i.e., borage oil, evening primrose oil)**
- **Fish (i.e., wild salmon, sardines)**
- **Avocados**

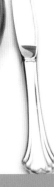

DO THIS TODAY

1 **Choose More Good Fat and Less Bad Fat**
Start keeping track of the Fat in your Fat Loss Plates (from dressings, sauces, cheese, etc.) – keep it to one Fatty Protein, or Fatty Fast Carb or single serving of Fat, and reduce the amount of Saturated Fat you eat (in pork and red meats, dairy and oil-based condiments). And, for the rest of your *21 Day Metabolism Makeover*, avoid breaded or fried foods and make sure you read every nutritional label so you can steer clear of ANY food containing hazardous Trans Fats.

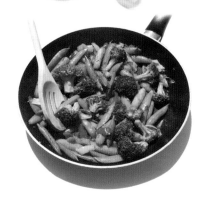

2 **Try Cooking With Less Fat**
It's much easier than you think to dramatically reduce the amount of high-calorie, metabolism-slowing fat in your favorite foods. Prove it to yourself today by cooking a reduced fat version of one of your favorite foods. Check out the tips on pages 22 to 25 of *How to Make a Fat Loss Plate* to learn how to lose the fat and keep the flavor in all your cooking.

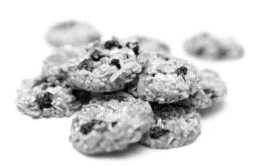

3 **Upgrade to Accelerator Snacks**
You've now made all the significant changes to the way that you are eating on the *21 Day Metabolism Makeover*. For the rest of the 21 days choose to eat ONLY Accelerator snacks as described in the Snack and Treat Guide. They will help jump start your metabolism the fastest, and keep you in the middle of Fat Burning zone all day long.

Today completes all the major food related tweaks for your *21 Day Metabolism Makeover*. You are now eating 100% on the plan, your metabolism is starting to run on high and you should be burning body fat at a tremendous rate!

DAY 6

EAT MORE HEALTHY FAT

Starting today, choose healthy fats instead of unhealthy Saturated Fats. Limit the fat in your Fat Loss Plates to one serving of Fatty Protein, Fatty Fast Carb, OR Fat, AND avoid any foods containing hazardous Trans Fats

✓ TO DO'S
(check when done)

- ☐ Listen to the **Day 6** Audio Program
- ☐ Substitute Healthy Fats for unhealthy fats in your meals
- ☐ Have only one serving of Fatty Protein, Fatty Fast Carb or Fat at each meal.
- ☐ Avoid Dangerous Trans Fats
- ☐ Eat Breakfast as soon as I get up
- ☐ Eat Fat Loss Meals & Accelerator Snacks every 2 to 3 hours
- ☐ Drink more water & avoid alcohol
- ☐ _____
- ☐ _____
- ☐ _____
- ☐ _____

TODAY'S CALLS

_____
_____
_____
_____
_____
_____

TODAY'S SCHEDULE

B-FAST / SNACK: Time   **Mins. Since Waking Up:** Time

I ate/drank:

EAT! Protein

7:00 am

8:00 am

9:00 am

B-FAST / SNACK: Time   **Hours Since Breakfast:** Time

I ate/drank:

EAT! Protein

10:00 am

11:00 am

12:00 pm

LUNCH / SNACK: Time   **Hours Since Snack:** Time

I ate/drank:

EAT! Protein

1:00 pm

2:00 pm

SNACK: Time   **Hours Since Lunch:** Time

I ate/drank:

EAT! Protein

EXERCISE ☐ YES ☐ NO   TIME [   ]

What/how much?

_____
_____

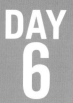

DID YOU KNOW...

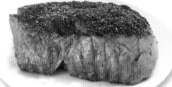

Some steaks
have MORE THAN
**100 grams of
Saturated Fat?**

TODAY'S SCHEDULE

3:00 pm

4:00 pm

5:00 pm

INNER: Time   **Hours Since Snack:** Time

te/drank:

EAT!

6:00 pm

7:00 pm

8:00 pm

NACK: Time   **Hours Since Dinner:** Time

te/drank:

EAT!

9:00 pm

0:00 pm

NACK: Time   **Hours Since Snack:** Time

te/drank:

EAT!

1:00 pm

Time I Went to Bed: Time

OUR FAVORITE FAT LOSS CONDIMENTS

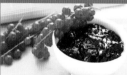

- Smuckers® Sugar Free Jams/Jellies
- St. Dalfour® Fruit Jam
- Knudsen® Light Sour Cream
- Follow Your Heart® Vegenaise
- Follow Your Heart® Spicy Southwestern Ranch Dressing
- Earth Balance® Whipped Buttery Spread
- Smart® Squeeze Nonfat Magarine Spread
- I Can't Believe It's Not Butter® Orginal Spray
- Horizon® Organic Unsalted Butter
- Smart Balance® Buttery Spread
- Tropical® Organic Strawberry Preserves Jelly
- Wild Mountain® Organic Honey
- French's® Mustard
- Maple Grove Farms®

NOTES

For each 8 oz. glass of water consumed, CIRCLE A NUMBER ➜ 1 2 3 4 5 6 7 8 9 10 11 12

You have now made all the significant changes to your eating habits that you are going to make for the rest of your *21 Day Metabolism Makeover* . Your metabolism should be starting to burn fat at a tremendous rate! Today we are going to amp it up even more with one incredibly simple change...

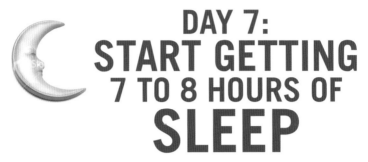

DAY 7:
START GETTING
7 TO 8 HOURS OF
SLEEP

You may feel like you can get by "just fine" on 4 or 5 hours of sleep but the fact of the matter is, study after study shows, your body NEEDS 7 to 8 hours of sleep to function properly. AND, if you don't get enough sleep it can cause you to *gain weight*. That's right—**those who don't get enough sleep may put on extra pounds!** Lack of sleep slows metabolism, increases cravings, and can reduce the benefits of exercise by not giving your body sufficient rest to recover. **So for the next 14 days, do whatever you have to do to get at least 7 hours of sleep each night**. Not only will this accelerate weight loss but you'll be amazed at how much better – and happier – you feel.

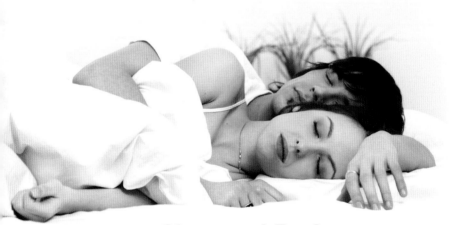

Sleep and Fat Loss

It may seem too simple to believe, but one of the best ways to lose weight is simply to get a few more hours of sleep. Study after study shows *a link between sleep deprivation and obesity*. In fact, several large scale studies in the United States and Europe suggest that the growing epidemic of obesity in our country may be partially due to the fact that people are getting less sleep.

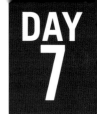

Getting too little sleep can affect your weight in a variety of ways. Sleep deprivation lowers the blood protein "leptin" which is responsible for suppressing appetite, while at the same time raising the level of "ghrelin," the substance that makes people want to eat. That means a craving or uncontrollable hunger may actually be due to lack of sleep. So next time you get one of those wild cravings for a sweet high-fat snack, ask yourself if you've been getting enough sleep. If not, try a 15 to 20 minute nap before you reach for the sweets.

Sleep deprivation also increases levels of cortisol, a stress hormone that increases blood sugar, interferes with the memory, retards muscle building, impairs your immune system and promotes abdominal fat! Also, studies involving subjects that were sleeping less than 8 hours per night indicated that physiologically they were decades older than they actually were!

Additionally, one study showed that sleep deprivation severely affects the body's ability to metabolize carbohydrates (glucose) – not only does that have dire consequences for weight loss but it can also lead to early stage type 2 diabetes.

It's a Big Deal...

This is nothing to take lightly. Even just a few hours less than the recommended 7 to 8 hours can have a huge impact on your weight. In the 1980's, the National Health and Nutrition Examination Survey (NHANES) found that people who got only 6 hours of sleep each night were 23% more likely to become obese than those who got 7 to 9 hours of sleep. And the less sleep you get the worse it gets. Those who got only 5 hours of sleep were 50% more likely to become obese and those who got 4 hours or less had a whopping 73% greater risk of becoming obese. So why make it harder on yourself. **Get the sleep you need**.

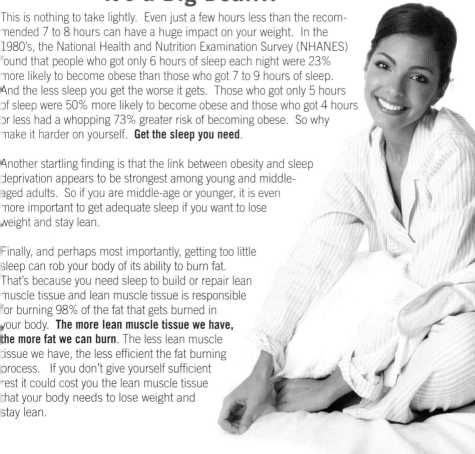

Another startling finding is that the link between obesity and sleep deprivation appears to be strongest among young and middle-aged adults. So if you are middle-age or younger, it is even more important to get adequate sleep if you want to lose weight and stay lean.

Finally, and perhaps most importantly, getting too little sleep can rob your body of its ability to burn fat. That's because you need sleep to build or repair lean muscle tissue and lean muscle tissue is responsible for burning 98% of the fat that gets burned in your body. **The more lean muscle tissue we have, the more fat we can burn**. The less lean muscle tissue we have, the less efficient the fat burning process. If you don't give yourself sufficient rest it could cost you the lean muscle tissue that your body needs to lose weight and stay lean.

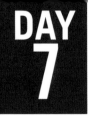

DAY 7

I'm a Busy Person...
I Don't Have Time to Sleep!

Our lives have gotten busier and busier and no one feels like they have enough time to sleep. But every aspect of life is better when you are well rested. **So you need to make YOU a priority**. The simplest way to get the sleep you need is to go to bed earlier. Start by turning in a half-hour earlier each night. Then when your body gets used to that, move your bedtime up another half-hour. Keep tweaking it until you are up to 7 to 8 hours a night.

If your schedule absolutely does not permit 7 to 8 straight hours of sleep, try to get 15 to 20 minute power-naps two or three times a day. In Japan they encourage napping during business hours as power-naps have been proven to help with mental concentration, alertness and proficiency. Anything you can do to give your body time to recover and reduce cortisol levels the better for your weight loss efforts.

But What If I Have Trouble Sleeping?

There are several strategies for coping with insomnia. One of the simplest is to start going to bed and **getting up at the same time every day**. Your body operates on cycles and gets used to them. Having a regular sleep pattern can help reduce insomnia and increase mental alertness during the day.

If you aren't exercising, adding exercise to your day is one of the best ways to improve the quantity and quality of your sleep. However, if sleeping is a problem, get your exercise earlier in the day as exercise will increase alertness so it could keep you up if you do it in the evening. Also avoid caffeine and nicotine 6 hours before bed time.

Whatever you do, find a way to get the extra hours of sleep in. **It could literally help you SLEEP THE POUNDS AWAY!**

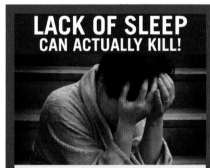

LACK OF SLEEP
CAN ACTUALLY KILL!

British Scientists, after studying more than 1000 civil servants over the course of eight years, found that those who got only 5 hours of sleep each night **DOUBLED** their chance of dying of a heart attack compared to those who got 7 hours of sleep. Those participants who deprived themselves of sleep were much more likely to develop cardiovascular problems and die prematurely. Most humans are programmed for about 7 hours of sleep says the author of the study. 7 to 8 hours seems to be the sweet spot. Interestingly, **TOO MUCH** sleep was just as dangerous: Those who slept more than 8 hours also died at twice the normal weight. So if you are sleeping too little, do yourself a favor and cut your risk of dying of a heart attack in half – **GO TO BED!**

DO THIS TODAY

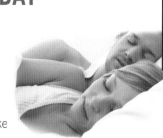

1 Get 7 to 8 Hours of Sleep Tonight

You're now eating in a way that absolutely *maximizes* your metabolism. Starting today you are going to increase your weight loss with one of the simplest activities possible – sleeping. Rearrange your schedule, or do whatever you need to do, to get to bed early tonight and make sure that you get 7 to 8 hours of sleep.

2 Start Journaling How Many Hours of Sleep You Get Each Day

Starting today, keep track of how many hours of sleep you get each night and record it in the space in the lower right hand portion of your planner pages. Then pay attention to how you feel on days where you've gotten a good night's sleep. How does it affect your mood? Cravings? Your weight loss? Look over your schedule for the next two weeks, figure out how you can get 7 to 8 hours in each night and schedule your bedtimes and wake times on your Planner Pages for the rest of the 21 days. Remember, for this *21 Day Metabolism Makeover* induction you want to get your metabolism burning fat as fast as possible and getting enough sleep is a critical component.

3 Reward Yourself and Set a New Weekly Goal

Congratulations! You've finished the first week of the program and are already well on your way to the lean and healthy body you've always wanted, so now it is time to reward yourself. Give yourself the reward you laid out on page 29 of the *Rapid Results Success Journal* and set your goal and reward for next week. (Remember, you're not going to weigh yourself until Day 21, so don't set next week's goals in terms of pounds lost.) You may choose to add 20 minutes of exercise each day this week, or follow through in an area where you stumbled last week. Whatever you think will best help you achieve your goal, write it down and set a reward that will help keep you motivated.

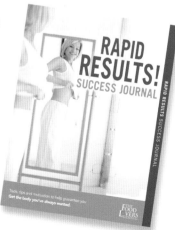

DAY 7

START GETTING
7 TO 8 HOURS OF SLEEP

Starting tonight, make sure you get 7 to 8 hours of sleep a night. This simple tweak will accelerate fat loss AND make you "feel" fantastic!

✓ TO DO'S
(check when done)

- ☐ Listen to the **Day 7** Audio Program
- ☐ Get 7 to 8 hours of sleep
- ☐ Reward yourself and set a new weekly goal
- ☐ Eat Breakfast as soon as I get up
- ☐ Eat Fat Loss Meals and Accelerator Snacks every 2 to 3 hours
- ☐ Drink more water & avoid alcohol
- ☐ Choose healthy fats & limit unhealthy fats
- ☐ _____
- ☐ _____
- ☐ _____
- ☐ _____

TODAY'S CALLS

_____
_____
_____
_____
_____
_____
_____

TODAY'S SCHEDULE

B-FAST / SNACK: Time ___   **Mins. Since Waking Up:** Time ___

I ate/drank: _____

EAT!

7:00 am

8:00 am

9:00 am

B-FAST / SNACK: Time ___   **Hours Since Breakfast:** Time ___

I ate/drank: _____

EAT!

10:00 am

11:00 am

12:00 pm

LUNCH / SNACK: Time ___   **Hours Since Snack:** Time ___

I ate/drank: _____

EAT!

1:00 pm

2:00 pm

SNACK: Time ___   **Hours Since Lunch:** Time ___

I ate/drank: _____

EAT!

EXERCISE   ☐ YES   ☐ NO   TIME [_____]

What/how much? _____

_____
_____

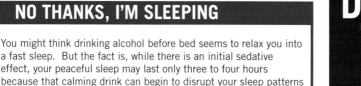

NO THANKS, I'M SLEEPING

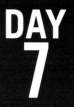

DAY
7

You might think drinking alcohol before bed seems to relax you into a fast sleep. But the fact is, while there is an initial sedative effect, your peaceful sleep may last only three to four hours because that calming drink can begin to disrupt your sleep patterns and actually increase the symptoms of sleep deprivation!

TODAY'S SCHEDULE

:00 pm _____

:00 pm _____

:00 pm _____

NNER: Time   **Hours Since Snack:** Time

te/drank:

AT!

:00 pm _____

:00 pm _____

:00 pm _____

NACK: Time   **Hours Since Dinner:** Time

te/drank:

AT!

:00 pm _____

:00 pm _____

NACK: Time   **Hours Since Snack:** Time

te/drank:

AT!

:00 pm _____

Time I Went to Bed: Time

FOODS THAT HELP YOU
SLEEP

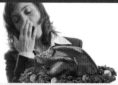

Foods that contain the amino acid **Tryptophan** contribute to restful sleep. **Tryptophan** is the amino acid that the body uses to make serotonin, the neurotransmitter that slows down nerve traffic so your brain isn't so busy. The following foods are high in the sleep-inducing amino acid **Tryptophan**:

- Poultry (Turkey!)
- Beans
- Rice
- Hummus
- Eggs
- Sesame seeds, sunflower seeds
- Dairy products: cottage cheese, cheese, milk
- Soy products: soy milk, tofu, soybean nuts
- Seafood

Remember a **lighter dinner** is more likely to give you a **restful night's sleep**.

NOTES

For each 8 oz. glass of water consumed, CIRCLE A NUMBER ➜ 1 2 3 4 5 6 7 8 9 10 11 12

w many hours did you sleep last night? _____

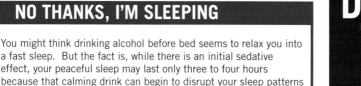

DAY 8

Just when you thought you had done everything you can do to rev up your metabolism and burn fat like never before – guess what? There is one simple technique that can **ACCELERATE YOUR METABOLISM** even more. By implementing fat burning cardio into your life you can dramatically speed up the process of reducing your waistline – and you can do it in very little time!

DAY 8: DO 12 MINUTES OF FAT BURNING CARDIO

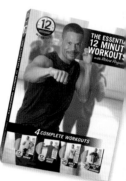

Starting today, you are going to take your body's fat burning processes to the next level by doing 12 minutes of fat burning cardio-respiratory exercise twice a week. You can simply pop in your *12 Minute Workout DVD* or do any other cardio activity -- walking, jogging, riding your bike or anything else you like as long as you are elevating your heart rate for at least 12 minutes. If you've already been exercising, that's great. Simply add 12 more minutes to the exercise you're already doing. Go for it! Just don't overdo it -- the goal is to start slow and work your way up so you are always increasing your workout and maximizing your results.

What is Fat Burning Cardio?

Cardio-respiratory (fat burning cardio) exercise is also known as aerobic exercise and it literally means to exercise "in oxygen." Strengthening your cardio-respiratory system means your lungs are better able to deliver oxygen to your bloodstream and muscles, which is critical to your body's ability to burn calories.

Generally, this type of exercise is performed at a moderate intensity for a sustained period of time. It is particularly important for strengthening your heart and lungs. Fat burning cardio can also help reduce the risk of coronary artery disease and help to lower blood pressure and cholesterol levels. Additionally, it makes you "feel" better. Not only are you less likely to get tired when you walk up the stairs or trot across the street, but you'll find that when you do this type of exercise regularly, you have more energy all day long and an increased sense of general "well-being."

Why is It Called Fat Burning?

While the single biggest component of weight loss is proper eating, cardio and resistance exercise are a close second, and they each have slightly different benefits. Cardio's short term benefit is simple. Performing cardio elevates your heart rate and that means you burn more calories. So every second you are doing cardio exercise you are burning more calories.

But there is a long term benefit to cardio exercise as well. Doing cardio workouts regularly enhances your body's ability to burn fat for energy both during the activity AND when resting (such as watching TV on the couch). That's because consistent performance of cardio increases your body's production of the enzyme "lipoprotein lpase," which breaks down fat into its component fatty acids. These fatty acids are released in the bloodstream and transported to your lean muscle tissue and other tissue where they are taken up by the cells, transferred into the mitochondria and broken down to release energy. The more cardio you do, the more of these powerful fat burning enzymes your body produces. And that means the more fit you become – the greater amounts of fat you can burn, whether you are simply walking or working out with greater intensity.

Why 12 Minutes?

Your body is always burning both fat and carbs for fuel; however, during an aerobic cardio workout once you reach the 12 minute mark (not counting cool down and warm up), there is a shift in body chemistry where your body begins producing fat burning enzymes at a higher rate. So whenever you are doing a cardio workout, you want to do at least 12 minutes. This optimizes your fat burning potential to give you the fastest results.

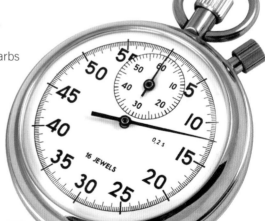

> **"The aerobic benefit is optimized when sustained for at least 12 minutes."**
> **Covert Baily, Author of *Fit or Fat***

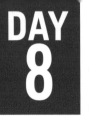

DAY 8

How Hard Should I Work?

At the beginning, it doesn't matter how hard you work. The important thing is that you get your heart rate elevated and keep it there for at least 12 minutes twice a week. Start at a pace where you are comfortable, then try to inch it up a bit each time. Go a bit faster or a bit farther. If you are working out with your *12 Minute Workout DVD*, just increase the intensity each time you do it – lift your legs a bit higher, or increase your pace with each workout. This baby-step approach is actually one of the most effective ways to get results because your body has a tendency to adapt to whatever activity you do, so by increasing your workout intensity just a bit each time, you can get the maximum benefit from each workout.

The "Talk Test"

You may have heard about a "target heart rate" where your body is burning the optimum amount of fat – it's also sometimes called the "fat burning zone." Well, it's real and one of the easiest ways to make sure you are in the "fat burning zone" is the "Talk Test." Ideally, you want to be working as hard as you can while still being able to carry on a conversation. So start your activity, then increase the intensity. Once you reach the point where you are starting to get out of breath, back down just a hair to where you can still talk. Once there, try to maintain this pace where you are going as fast or hard as you can but can still talk normally, and you will be in your "target heart rate" zone. The great thing about this method is it adapts as you do. As you get in better shape, you will be able to go a bit faster and a bit harder and still be able to carry on a normal conversation. This is ideal because as you get more fit you'll **need** to work a bit harder to stay in the "fat burning zone". So the "Talk Test" will work for you no matter what level you are at.

Scheduling Your Fat Burning

The number one reason people give for not exercising is that they "don't have the time." But think about this: there are 168 hours in a week and right now all you need to do is find a total of 24 minutes each week – for **significant** results!

The best way to make sure you do your cardio routine regularly is to schedule it. Look ahead in your Planner Pages and pick a time when you can fit in 12 minutes of fat burning. Decide whether it will be first thing in the morning, during lunch or after work. Then schedule it just like you would a doctor's appointment. Treat this scheduled appointment with the same respect and importance you give to your other appointments. Getting lean, healthy and happy are the most important things in your life so make your appointments for achieving those goals a top priority.

DO THIS TODAY

1 **Do 12 Minutes of Fat Burning Cardio Exercise**
Today you are going to amplify the fat loss results that all the changes to your eating are providing by adding 12 minutes of Fat Burning Cardio. Either pop in your *12 Minute Workout DVD* or do some other cardiovascular activity that keeps your heart rate elevated for at least 12 consecutive minutes. Then go through your Planner Pages, decide what time of day you can find time to burn some fat and schedule your cardio workouts for two times a week for the rest of your *21 Day Metabolism Makeover*.

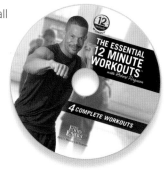

2 **Start Paying Attention to How You FEEL**
Food is the fuel your body runs on. The higher the quality of fuel you put into it, the better it will run. Now that you have made all the changes you're going to be making to your eating habits and have fully optimized your metabolism, start to pay attention to how you feel as you go through today and the next 13 days on the plan. How is your energy level throughout the day? How are you sleeping? How do you feel when you wake up? Jot these things down on your Planner Pages, then review them at the end of each week and see how it is related to what you ate or what exercise you did. You'll be surprised at what an effect healthy eating and exercise can have on your mood, your health and your happiness.

DAY 8

DO 12 MINUTES OF
FAT BURNING CARDIO EXERCISE

Starting today, take your fat burning to the next level by doing 12 minutes of Fat Burning Cardio twice a week. Do your *12 Minute Workout DVD* or any cardio activity you enjoy as long as you keep you heart rate elevated for at least 12 consecutive minutes.

✓ TO DO'S
(check when done)

- ☐ Listen to the **Day 8** Audio Program
- ☐ Do 12 minutes of Fat Burning Cardio exercise
- ☐ Get 7 to 8 hours of sleep
- ☐ Eat Breakfast as soon as I get up
- ☐ Eat Fat Loss Meals and Accelerator Snacks every 2 to 3 hours
- ☐ Drink more water and avoid alcohol
- ☐ Choose only healthy breads and sweets
- ☐ Pay attention to my Fat intake
- ☐ _____
- ☐ _____
- ☐ _____
- ☐ _____

TODAY'S CALLS

_____
_____
_____
_____
_____
_____

TODAY'S SCHEDULE

B-FAST / SNACK: Time   **Mins. Since Waking Up:** Time
I ate/drank:

EAT!

7:00 am

8:00 am

9:00 am

B-FAST / SNACK: Time   **Hours Since Breakfast:** Time
I ate/drank:

EAT!

10:00 am

11:00 am

12:00 pm

LUNCH / SNACK: Time   **Hours Since Snack:** Time
I ate/drank:

EAT!

1:00 pm

2:00 pm

SNACK: Time   **Hours Since Lunch:** Time
I ate/drank:

EAT!

EXERCISE ☐ YES ☐ NO   TIME ☐

What/how much?

_____
_____

SING YOUR WAY TO A REDUCED WAISTLINE

When performing your cardio fat burning routine, test yourself and see if you can sing in one breath: "Twinkle, twinkle little star, how I wonder what you are." If you can't say "Twinkle, twinkle little star" in one breath – slow down because you are working too hard. If you can get all the way through to "what you are," pump it up a bit. If you are at your "target heart rate" you'll run out of breath somewhere through the second half of the line.

TODAY'S SCHEDULE

3:00 pm

4:00 pm

5:00 pm

DINNER: Time   **Hours Since Snack:** Time

te/drank:

EAT!

6:00 pm

7:00 pm

8:00 pm

SNACK: Time   **Hours Since Dinner:** Time

te/drank:

EAT!

9:00 pm

10:00 pm

SNACK: Time   **Hours Since Snack:** Time

te/drank:

EAT!

11:00 pm

Time I Went to Bed: Time

5 KEYS TO EXERCISE SUCCESS

1 Choose a **convenient time** of the day to exercise.

Make sure you are ready and *commit* to following through.

2 Wear **comfortable clothes** that allow a full range of motion.

It's also important to wear clothing that allows the body to ventilate.

3 Wear **supportive athletic shoes** with a molded sole and plenty of traction.

"Cross Trainer" shoes are a good example.

4 Make sure you have an open space where you will be exercising.

If indoors, you don't want to hurt yourself or cause damage.

5 Have a water bottle with you at all times.

Hydration is extremely important!

NOTES

For each 8 oz. glass of water consumed, CIRCLE A NUMBER ➜ 1 2 3 4 5 6 7 8 9 10 11 12

ow many hours did you sleep last night? _____

DAY 9

Now that you are eating Fat Loss Meals and Fat Loss Snacks throughout the day, drinking plenty of water and scheduling opportunities for fat burning exercise, it's time to **OPTIMIZE YOUR METABOLISM** – and your general health – with additional nutrients.

DAY 9: OPTIMIZE YOUR METABOLISM
WITH NUTRITIONAL SUPPLEMENTS

The healthier you are, the more efficiently your metabolism works. The more efficiently your metabolism works, the easier it is for you to burn fat. Nutritional supplements are a great way to ensure that you are getting all the nutrients you need to keep your body healthy and burning fat as fast as possible. **So starting today, add a high-quality multi-vitamin to your day**. Additionally, read over the list of recommended supplements, **The Fat Loss 5**, and choose the ones you want to use to optimize your metabolism and add them to your daily regimen.

Is a Multi-Vitamin Really Important?

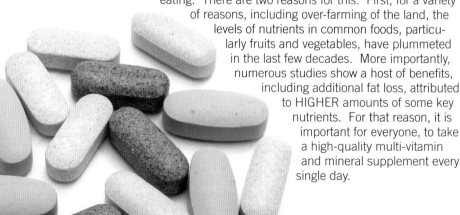

While you are now eating in a much more healthy manner, you still may not be getting "optimum" amounts of the nutrients your body needs from the food you are eating. There are two reasons for this. First, for a variety of reasons, including over-farming of the land, the levels of nutrients in common foods, particularly fruits and vegetables, have plummeted in the last few decades. More importantly, numerous studies show a host of benefits, including additional fat loss, attributed to HIGHER amounts of some key nutrients. For that reason, it is important for everyone, to take a high-quality multi-vitamin and mineral supplement every single day.

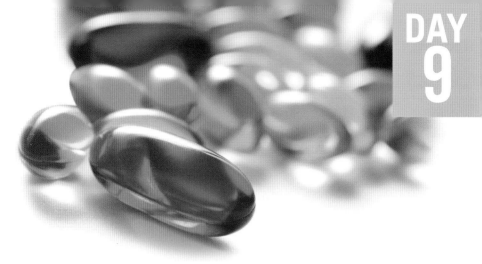

Which Multi Should I Take?

Just like choosing foods, it begins with reading the label. And remember, always check with your doctor before taking any supplements.

Things to look for:

- **Look for "USP" on a label.** This specifies that the supplement meets the standards of the U.S. Pharmacopoeia.
- **Carefully read specialized formulas (those for women, men, seniors, etc.).** Claims on nutritional supplements aren't regulated like prescription drugs (or even foods); each company sets its own standards. For example, "women's" formulas have additional calcium, but may lack the Daily Value for Vitamin D, which is necessary for proper calcium absorption.
- **Check the expiration date!**
- **Check out the levels of each vitamin and mineral.** Look for 100% of the Daily Value for Vitamins B1 (thiamin), B2 (riboflavin), Niacin, Vitamin B6, B12, C, D, E, and Folic Acid. Often once-daily vitamin formulas do NOT include the full 100% daily recommendation of key antioxidants, like Vitamin C and E, so you may need to take supplements of these critical nutrients separately.
- **Check the serving size.** Some minerals like calcium are very large, and you may need to take up to six tablets daily to get the Recommended Daily Allowance.
- **Skip the iron in a multi-vitamin.** For cancer patients, it is advisable to ask your medical team about whether or not you should take iron in a multi-vitamin. Unless you have iron-deficient anemia, are at risk of anemia or have had recent surgery, you may not need additional iron. Also, iron supplements can cause constipation, so you will need to increase your fiber and fluid intake.
- **Take with food.** It is generally best to take multi-vitamins with food to assist with absorption. Supplements are available in liquid form as well as chewable tablets for those with problems swallowing capsules or tablets.
- **Check out our website.** We'll post links to our favorite "Multi's" including research, guidelines and recommendations for achieving "optimum health" with higher levels of key vitamins, minerals and other types of supplements.

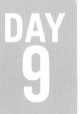

DAY 9

THE FAT LOSS 5

As you may have seen at your local drugstore, there are dozens and dozens of supplements available for purchase. Your Food Lovers experts have reviewed these options, and have carefully handpicked a few of the most valuable supplements. This daily regimen, known as **The Fat Loss 5**, includes key supplements that support an increase in your body's ability to burn fat as well as accelerate your metabolism.

THE FAT LOSS 5

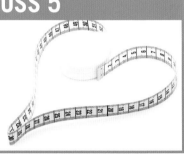

1 Borage Oil
2 Omega-3 Fatty Acids (Fish Oil)
3 Ground Flaxseed
4 Protein Powder
5 5 Way Metabolic Fat Fighter

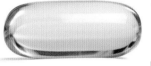

1 **Borage Oil** is a rich source of gamma-linolenic acid which has a unique ability to discourage fat storage, encourage the use of stored fat for energy, and rev up your metabolism. Research has shown that the gamma-linolenic acid in borage oil activates a metabolic process that can burn close to 50% of the body's total calories. In one gamma-linolenic acid study, individuals lost from 9.6 to 11.4 pounds over a six week period. Other sources of gamma-linolenic acid are black currant oil and evening primose oil.

Recommended Dosage
- **For weight loss**: 1000 mg./day.
- **For general health when not losing weight**: 250 to 500 mg./day.

2 **Omega-3 Fatty Acids** (in the form of Fish Oil) are associated with decreased fat storage, a reduction in heart disease and also known for their potential to enhance insulin sensitivity. Essential Fatty Acid deficiency has also been tied to low leptin levels. Leptin is a hormone that regulates our appetite. By supplementing your nutrition habits with Essential Fatty Acids such as Omega-3, you may be better able to control your appetite and burn more fat.

Recommended Dosage
- **For weight loss**: 1 gram/day on days you don't eat fish.
- **For those with high triglycerides**: 2 to 4 grams/day.
- **For those with rheumatoid arthritis, psoriasis, or other auto-immune disorders**: 3 grams/day.

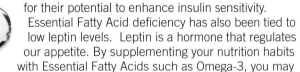

❸ Ground Flaxseed is a rich source of lignans, soluble and insoluble fiber, protein, vitamins, minerals and the truest source of alpha-linolenic acid.

This Essential Fatty Acid aids in stabilizing blood sugar and helps to boost metabolism. It's a natural way for you to increase your energy, accelerate your metabolism, control appetite, drop unwanted inches and shed pounds.

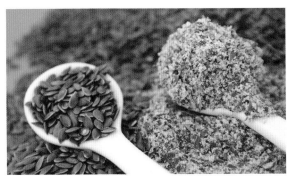

Ground flaxseed has a delicious nutty flavor and is delicious sprinkled on cereal, salad, yogurt, and fruit. Or it can be mixed with water, juice, or blended into a tasty smoothie. You can also bake ground flaxseed into cookies, muffins and bread.

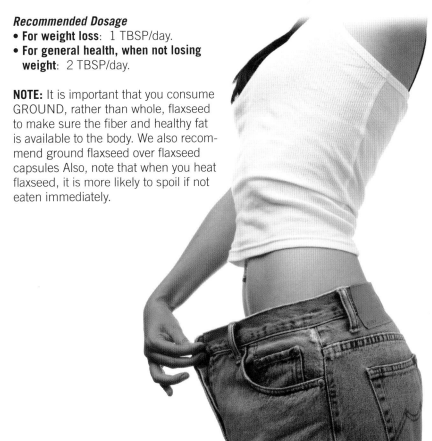

Recommended Dosage
- **For weight loss**: 1 TBSP/day.
- **For general health, when not losing weight**: 2 TBSP/day.

NOTE: It is important that you consume GROUND, rather than whole, flaxseed to make sure the fiber and healthy fat is available to the body. We also recommend ground flaxseed over flaxseed capsules Also, note that when you heat flaxseed, it is more likely to spoil if not eaten immediately.

4 Protein Powder. While protein powder is not always grouped with these kinds of nutritional supplements, due to the fat loss benefits associated with increasing protein intake, it can be a helpful addition to your daily eating.

There is convincing evidence that a higher protein intake increases thermogenesis (the amount of calories your body burns as a result of consumption, digestion and absorption) and satiety compared to nutrition habits with lower protein content. Additionally, because the chief calorie burner of your metabolism (lean muscle tissue) is made up of protein, having an adequate amount of protein readily available increases the potential for your body to build and repair your all-important lean muscle tissue.

High-quality protein powder is one of the best ways to ensure that you maximize your lean protein intake without adding unwanted fats and sugars. When choosing a protein powder, look for the following guidelines, in order to achieve the healthiest weight loss:

- 100% Whey Protein
- A yield of 15-25g of Protein per serving
- No sugar and extremely low carb – 3g total carb or less
- Less than 2g of Fat per serving

Note: In many of the recipes found in *The Love to Eat Cookbook*, *Million Meals Menu Planner*, *Classic Comfort Food Recipe Cards* (specifically our smoothie and celebrated pancake recipe and many of our muffin recipes), protein powder is a key ingredient and is used in place of flour.

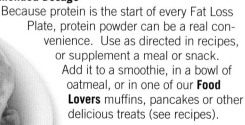

Recommended Dosage

Because protein is the start of every Fat Loss Plate, protein powder can be a real convenience. Use as directed in recipes, or supplement a meal or snack. Add it to a smoothie, in a bowl of oatmeal, or in one of our **Food Lovers** muffins, pancakes or other delicious treats (see recipes).

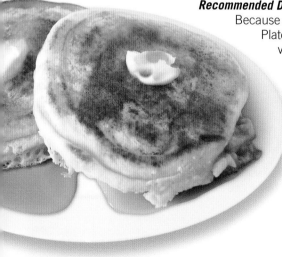

5 **5 Way Metabolic Fat Fighter**: Finally, for fastest fat loss results Robert Ferguson recommends the **5 Way Metabolic Fat Fighter** from Provida Labs. This Ephedra-free supplement is a scientific blend of the most effective herbs and nutrients including Chromium Picolinate, ECGC, Guarana, Green Tea Extract, Calcium and a full complement of critical B-complex vitamins that work together to help naturally accelerate your metabolism and aid in fat loss 5 different ways:

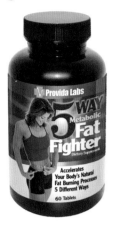

1 Helps Increase Metabolism to Burn More Calories

2 Helps Accelerate Conversion of Food to Energy

3 Helps Convert Stored Fat to Energy

4 Helps Burn Carbs as Energy Instead of Storing Them as Fat

5 Increases Energy to Burn More Calories

Recommended Dosage: 2 to 4 Tablets / Day with meals. See label for additional instructions.

DO THIS TODAY

1 Start Taking A Multi-Vitamin

Now that you are eating in a way that fully accelerates your metabolism – three Fat Loss Meals plus snacks every two to three hours – it is time to further optimize your fat loss processes by adding a multi-vitamin to your routine. Choose a high-quality multi-vitamin/mineral supplement and start taking it each day with breakfast to make sure you are getting all the nutrition you need to keep your body burning fat as fast as possible.

2 Start Journaling Your Nutritional Supplements

Review **The Fat Loss 5**, decide which of those supplements you are going to use to accelerate your results and then stock up! You'll notice that your Planner Pages now include a line at the lower right to journal all the nutritional supplements you take. So starting today, write down all the vitamins, minerals, and other supplements you take, including protein powder, in your Planner Pages so you can start to see the relationship between nutritional supplementation and fat loss.

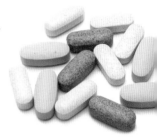

NOTES

1 For each 8 oz. glass of water consumed, CIRCLE A NUMBER ➔ 1 2

How many hours did you sleep last night? _8 hrs_

Supplements I took today? _1000 mgs Borage Oil, Groun_

21 DAY METABOLISM MAKEOV

DAY 9

OPTIMIZE YOUR METABOLISM
WITH NUTRITIONAL SUPPLEMENTS

Starting today, make sure your body is getting all the nutrients it needs to burn fat as fast as possible by taking a high-quality multi-vitamin mineral supplement. Also review **The Fat Loss 5** and stock up on the nutrients you want to use to accelerate fat loss.

✓ TO DO'S
(check when done)

- [ ] Listen to the **Day 9** Audio Program
- [ ] Take a multi-vitamin mineral supplement
- [ ] Start taking some or all of **The Fat Loss 5**
- [ ] Get 7 to 8 hours of sleep
- [ ] Eat Breakfast as soon as I get up
- [ ] Eat Fat Loss Meals and Accelerator Snacks every 2 to 3 hours
- [ ] Choose only healthy breads and sweets
- [ ] Drink more water and avoid alcohol
- [ ] _____
- [ ] _____
- [ ] _____
- [ ] _____

TODAY'S CALLS

_____
_____
_____
_____
_____
_____
_____

TODAY'S SCHEDULE

B-FAST / SNACK: Time   **Mins. Since Waking Up:** Time
I ate/drank:

EAT! Protein

7:00 am

8:00 am

9:00 am

B-FAST / SNACK: Time   **Hours Since Breakfast:** Time
I ate/drank:

EAT! Protein

10:00 am

11:00 am

12:00 pm

LUNCH / SNACK: Time   **Hours Since Snack:** Time
I ate/drank:

EAT! Protein

1:00 pm

2:00 pm

SNACK: Time   **Hours Since Lunch:** Time
I ate/drank:

EAT! Protein

EXERCISE ☐ YES ☐ NO   **TIME** _____
What/how much?
_____
_____

CALCIUM

Calcium is tremendously important for bone strength and health. **Multiple studies show an increase in Bone Mass Density with supplementation of 1000 mg. taken daily.** While that level is the RDA (%DV), the leading multivitamin contains 162 mg. or only 16% of that optimum amount.

TODAY'S SCHEDULE

3:00 pm

4:00 pm

5:00 pm

DINNER: Time   **Hours Since Snack:** Time

ate/drank:

EAT!

6:00 pm

7:00 pm

8:00 pm

SNACK: Time   **Hours Since Dinner:** Time

ate/drank:

EAT!

9:00 pm

10:00 pm

SNACK: Time   **Hours Since Snack:** Time

ate/drank:

EAT!

11:00 pm

Time I Went to Bed: Time

READ THE SUPPLEMENT FACTS

Most grocery store supplements are based on the Recommended Daily Allowance (RDA – now updated to "% Daily Value" or "%DV") which was created in the 1940's to help prevent end-stage diseases like scurvy and rickets. In other words, the RDA was designed to prevent nutritional deficiencies that were so serious they could lead to death. They were never designed to help create optimum health.

Since the RDA was created more than 50 years ago, there have been literally thousands of scientific studies documenting the remarkable benefits of certain vitamins and minerals – ranging from helping to prevent cancer and cardiovascular disease, improving immune system response and helping you live a longer, healthier life -- all from significantly higher dosage levels of certain nutrients than those established six decades ago.

For example, a four year study in the U.S. showed that 200 mcg a day of the mineral Selenium (nearly three times higher than the RDA of 70 mcg) resulted in a 45% reduction in lung cancer, 58% reduction in colorectal cancer and a 63% reduction in prostate cancer

Go to our website or www.ProvidaLabs.com for more information on optimum nutrition.

NOTES

For each 8 oz. glass of water consumed, CIRCLE A NUMBER ➔ 1 2 3 4 5 6 7 8 9 10 11 12

How many hours did you sleep last night? _____

Supplements I took today? _____

DAY 10

Now that you are eating and exercising in a way that has your metabolism racing, it's time to start making some other small changes that will make it easier to **stay lean and healthy for the rest of your life.**

DAY 10: STOCK YOUR CUPBOARDS AND PANTRY WITH FOOD LOVERS FOOD

Today, you are going to go grocery shopping and you are going to stock your kitchen with the very best foods, packaged goods and ingredients for fat loss. You'll start by evaluating the foods currently taking up space in your cupboards, pantry, and fridge. Then check the labels and look for the biggest enemies of fat loss:

1. Partially hydrogenated oils and fractionated oils
2. High fructose corn syrup and other refined sugars
3. White, bleached, and enriched flour
4. High levels of fat

Then head to the store and replace them with healthier versions that you love just as much that will cause your body to lose weight rather than gain it.

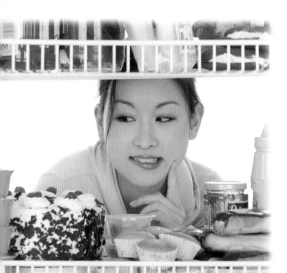

Stay in Control

Now that you're eating every 2 to 3 hours and keeping your metabolism burning its hottest, you are going to find that you are truly hungry when it's time to eat. When that healthy hunger appears, the last thing you want is to open up your pantry only to find that you lack the healthy fuel (food) necessary to keep your metabolism burning fat as fast as possible.

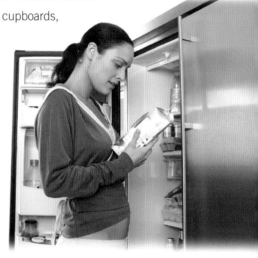

In fact, it is absolutely critical to keep good food on hand or you are almost certain to turn to something that will slow or stop fat loss. That is because, once your metabolism gets going and your body is burning all the food you eat every 2 to 3 hours your body will NEED to eat every 2 to 3 hours. Your hunger will grow and a physiological chain of events will take place that will force your body to take the shortest path to the sugar it needs for energy – by reaching for the highly-refined, junk food that can sabotage your efforts. It won't be your fault. This is a **physiological** pitfall that can overwhelm even the most disciplined soul and sabotage even the most diligent efforts.

The best way to avoid this is to clear out the worst enemies of fat loss and stock your cupboards with healthy fat-burning replacements – ones that you love!

Step 1: Evaluate Your Kitchen

Go through your entire kitchen - your pantry, cupboards, refrigerator and freezer and look at <u>everything</u>. Read the nutrition labels, apply all your Label Detective skills and look for products that will slow fat loss (i.e. products loaded with refined sugars, processed flours and hidden fats). Once you've identified those products that don't support an accelerated metabolism, get them out of your house. Toss them or give them away – but get rid of them! Then make a list of each and every food you threw away so you can find comparable products that are made with metabolism-friendly ingredients.

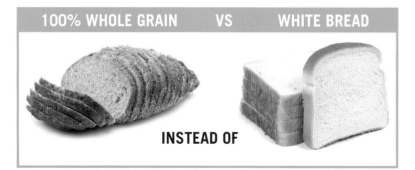

100% WHOLE GRAIN   VS   WHITE BREAD

INSTEAD OF

EXAMPLE: If you have bread in your pantry that is made with white flour – **DON'T PANIC** – we are not saying to eliminate bread from your kitchen. Continue eating bread but choose a brand of bread that is made with 100% whole wheat and less sugar. It's liable to have more flavor too!

Step 2: Make a Shopping List

Use the list on the following page as a starting place. We've made a list of staples that every healthy house will want to keep on-hand that will ensure you always have supplies to prepare Fat Loss Meals in minutes. Now we want you to supplement the list with your favorite foods:

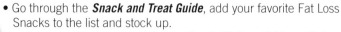

- Go through the *Snack and Treat Guide*, add your favorite Fat Loss Snacks to the list and stock up.
  - Review your notes in *How to Make a Fat Loss Plate* and add the ingredients to make your favorite Fat Loss Breakfasts, Lunches and Dinners.
    - Check out the *Classic Comfort Food Recipe Cards* and *The Love to Eat Cookbook* for more recipes and lists of fat burning substitutes for common ingredients.

As you go through the program you'll see that you can find a healthy alternative for each and every one of your favorite foods that will support the fat burning process. The goal is for you to continue eating all your favorite foods but discover alternative brands that support your revved-up metabolism. Once you have your list (don't put off till tomorrow what you can do today) go grocery shopping! Take a friend with you and make it fun!

MEAT SECTION

- Chicken Breast
- Lean Ground Turkey Breast
- Lean Deli Meats
- Fish
- _____
- _____
- _____
- _____
- _____
- _____
- _____
- _____
- _____
- _____
- _____
- _____

PRODUCE SECTION

- Potatoes
- Onions
- Bell Peppers
- Mushrooms
- Sweet Potatoes
- Avocado
- Tomatoes
- Apples
- Bananas
- Berries
- _____
- _____
- _____
- _____
- _____
- _____

DAIRY SECTION

- Skim Milk
- Low-Fat or Non-Fat Yogurt
- Low-Fat Cheesesticks
- Eggs or Egg Beaters
- _____
- _____
- _____
- _____
- _____
- _____
- _____
- _____
- _____

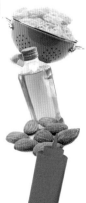

BREAKFAST AISLE

- Old-Fashioned Oatmeal
- Optimum Power Blueberry Cinnamon from Nature's Path
- _____
- _____
- _____
- _____
- _____
- _____
- _____
- _____
- _____

BREADS

- 100% Whole Wheat Bread,
- Whole Wheat Tortillas (*La Tortilla Factory*)
- _____
- _____
- _____
- _____
- _____
- _____
- _____
- _____

CANNED GOODS

- No Salt Added Beans
- No Salt Added Tomato Sauce
- No Salt Added Veggies
- Tuna Packed in Water
- _____
- _____
- _____
- _____
- _____
- _____

STAPLES

- Brown Rice/Wild Rice
- Whole Grain Pasta
- 100% Whole Wheat Flour
- Splenda
- Extra Virgin Olive Oil
- Grape Seed Oil
- Low Sodium Beef & Chicken Broth
- _____
- _____
- _____
- _____
- _____
- _____

CONDIMENTS & SPICES

- Salt-Free *Mrs. Dash* and *McCormick's* flavors
- No Salt Added Salsa
- All Natural Peanut Butter
- 100% Fruit Jam
- Fruit-Sweetened Ketchup
- Mustard
- *Newman's Own* or *Annie's Naturals* Salad Dressing
- _____
- _____
- _____
- _____

ADDITIONAL ITEMS

- Nuts (Almonds, Walnuts, etc)
- _____
- _____
- _____
- _____
- _____
- _____
- _____
- _____
- _____
- _____

DAY 10

SODIUM
THE OVERLOOKED "ENEMY OF FAT LOSS"

You've already made all the big changes to the way you're eating that will maximize your metabolism for the first 21 days. However, there is one last way you can DRAMATICALLY accelerate your weight loss results during this period and that is by paying attention to the amount of sodium you consume.

Sodium is an element most often found in salt (Sodium Chloride) and it is absolutely critical for your body to function properly. Without enough salt we would die. On the other hand, too much salt can have some dire consequences for your health AND your efforts to lose weight. Too much sodium can increase blood pressure, cause water retention and bloating (which results in weight gain) and generally slow the weight loss process. To make matters worse, restaurant meals and pre-packaged foods (and low fat and diet foods can be some of the worst offenders) are so loaded with sodium that it's not uncommon for the average person to consume 5 to 7 times the Recommended Daily Allowance. (The US Government recommends no more than 2300 mgs, most scientists suggest we only consume 500 mgs yet most people consume more than 6000 mgs/day.)

Like sugar, sodium hides under many different names:
1. Sodium Chloride (Table Salt)
2. Disodium Phosphate
3. Monosodium Glutamate (MSG)

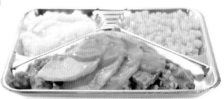

BEWARE of Sodium's Most Common Hiding Places:
1. Fast Foods – sandwiches, fries, etc.
2. Snack Foods – potato chips, pretzels, nuts, etc.
3. Processed Meats – sausages, hot dogs, lunch meats, etc.
4. Canned Vegetables and Soups
5. Dehydrated or Packaged Foods – "instant" meals and side dishes – soups, pastas & rice dishes, etc.
6. Sauces and Condiments – tomato sauce, hot sauce, soy sauce, etc.
7. White Bread and Rolls
8. Dairy Products
9. Frozen Entrees

Check labels because sodium content is always listed. And, try to choose "whole" foods over "packaged" or prepared foods – natural foods always have less Sodium. Finally, try to avoid adding salt to your food – there are a host of salt-free seasonings that taste great (see *The Love to Eat Cookbook*). For fastest fat loss results, **keep your Sodium intake below 700 mgs at any one meal**.

DO THIS TODAY

1 **Upgrade Your Pantry**
Go through your pantry, cupboards, and fridge. Clear out the biggest enemies of fat loss then go to the grocery store and stock your cupboards and fridge with your favorite fat burning foods.

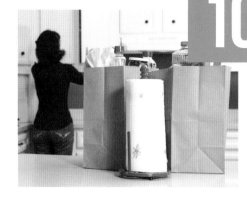

2 **Accelerate Your Results by Reducing Sodium Intake**
If you are used to adding salt to your food, for the rest of your *21 Day Metabolism Makeover* use half as much. If you can manage, skip it altogether and instead *try sodium-free seasonings like Mrs. Dash, McCormick's* or other seasonings like fresh ground pepper, garlic powder and fresh herbs. Doing this helps you keep from retaining water and feeling bloated. Also, check the labels on pre-packaged foods and *try to keep sodium to less than 700 mgs in a single meal*. It's not uncommon for a frozen entrée to have more than 1,000 mg of sodium in a single serving.

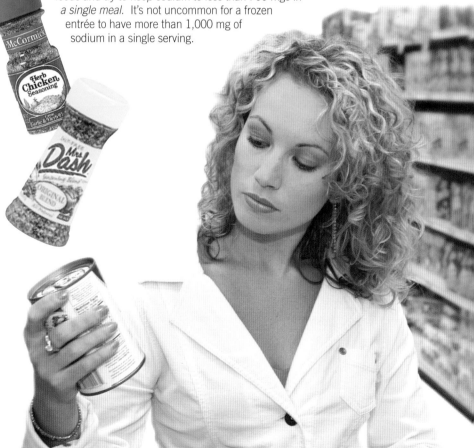

DAY 10

Day: ✓ [S] [M] [T] [W] [TH] [F] [S]   Date: ___ / ___ / ___

STOCK YOUR CUPBOARDS AND PANTRY
WITH FOOD LOVERS FOOD

Go grocery shopping and stock your kitchen with the very best foods, packaged goods and ingredients for fat loss. Start by evaluating the foods currently filling your pantry and fridge. Check the labels, look for the biggest "Enemies of Fat Los and then head to the store and replace them with healthier versions that you love just as much but which will cause your body to lose weight rather than gain it.

✓ TO DO'S
(check when done)

- ☐ Listen to the **Day 10** Audio Program
- ☐ Go grocery shopping and upgrade my pantry and fridge
- ☐ Do 12 minutes of Fat Burning Cardio exercise
- ☐ Take my nutritional supplements
- ☐ Get 7 to 8 hours of sleep
- ☐ Eat Fat Loss Meals and Accelerator Snacks every 2 to 3 hours
- ☐ Choose only healthy breads, sweets and Snacks
- ☐ Drink more water and avoid alcohol
- ☐ _____
- ☐ _____
- ☐ _____
- ☐ _____

TODAY'S CALLS

_____
_____
_____
_____
_____
_____

TODAY'S SCHEDULE

B-FAST / SNACK: Time   **Mins. Since Waking Up:** Time

I ate/drank:

EAT!

7:00 am

8:00 am

9:00 am

B-FAST / SNACK: Time   **Hours Since Breakfast:** Time

I ate/drank:

EAT!

10:00 am

11:00 am

12:00 pm

LUNCH / SNACK: Time   **Hours Since Snack:** Time

I ate/drank:

EAT!

1:00 pm

2:00 pm

SNACK: Time   **Hours Since Lunch:** Time

I ate/drank:

EAT!

EXERCISE   ☐ YES   ☐ NO   TIME [_____]

What/how much?

_____
_____

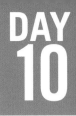

SODIUM - HOW EASILY IT HIDES

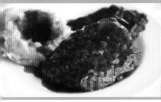

This restaurant meal has 2720 mgs of sodium. The USDA recommends **2300 mgs for the WHOLE DAY!**

TODAY'S SCHEDULE

3:00 pm

4:00 pm

5:00 pm

DINNER: Time   **Hours Since Snack:** Time

ate/drank:

EAT!

6:00 pm

7:00 pm

8:00 pm

SNACK: Time   **Hours Since Dinner:** Time

ate/drank:

EAT!

9:00 pm

10:00 pm

SNACK: Time   **Hours Since Snack:** Time

ate/drank:

EAT!

11:00 pm

Time I Went to Bed: Time

OUR FAVORITE SODIUM FREE SEASONINGS

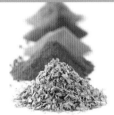

Make sure you check out pages 14 to 17 in *The Love to Eat Cookbook*. You'll find an extensive list of "Blah Busters" to fabulously liven up your dishes without added sodium. In addition to pure herbs and spices, a number of manufacturers offer no-sodium seasonings. We've found particularly tasty flavors from:

- **The Spice Hunter®**
- **McCormick®**
- **Frontier®**
- **Spike®**
- **Veg-It®**
- **Mrs. Dash®**

Spend a few moments perusing your grocery's spice aisle. New flavors are frequently added!

NOTES

For each 8 oz. glass of water consumed, CIRCLE A NUMBER ➜ 1 2 3 4 5 6 7 8 9 10 11 12

How many hours did you sleep last night? _____

Supplements I took today? _____

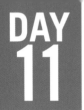

With **Food Lovers** you don't just lose the weight, you keep it off! And that's because you don't have to deprive yourself of **ANYTHING.** You really can eat **ALL** your family's favorite foods in a way that will cause you to lose weight and today you are going to **PROVE** it to yourself.

DAY 11:
TURN YOUR FAMILY'S FAVORITE MEAL INTO A
FAT LOSS PLATE

You've already learned how making small modifications to the <u>way</u> you prepare your food and how by selecting the right ingredients, you can make a HUGE impact on fat loss. Now, you are going to put it to the ultimate test by taking your family's favorite meal - meatloaf and mashed potatoes, lasagna, tacos, whatever they love best - and turning it into a fat burning Fat Loss Plate. **Use your knowledge of healthy ingredients and the tips in the first chapters of *The Love to Eat Cookbook* to tweak your recipe, then serve it up in the portions of a Fat Loss Plate**.

Learn to Eat to Be Lean FOREVER!

It's easy to get into a rut with what you are eating. You may have found two or three recipes you really like and you eat them several times a week because "it's easy." It's a common habit to fall into, but it can be dangerous for long term fat loss.

One of the major reasons that people fail at "diets" is because they get bored. If you feel limited by your choices, you'll get bored too. Think about it: are you still going to love those three "easy" meals if you're still eating them every week a year from now?

What makes **Food Lovers** different is that there are no limitations. You can turn anything you love into a Fat Loss Plate or Snack (with just a few small tweaks) and this is the day to prove it to yourself.

So today you are going to make sure you truly "love" what you eat and prove to yourself that you really can eat ANYTHING in a way that causes you to lose weight, be healthy and stay lean.

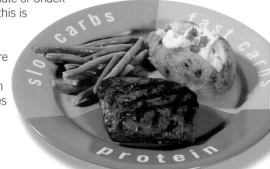

Mix it Up

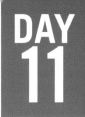

DAY 11

Today is the day to mix it up. If you've been eating the same Fat Loss Meals over and over or the same snacks every day, then, today, try something different. Over the next week try to **find three _new_ Fat Loss Meals** and **several _new_ snacks** that you love. And tonight, cook something that your family loves that **you haven't eaten since you started the program**. The more you love the food you are eating the easier it will be to keep eating that way and stay lean.

It's as Easy as... Pie!

Most families' favorite meals aren't that far off from the proportions of a Fat Loss Plate just as they are. They probably already include a **Protein**, a **Fast Carb** and a **Slow Carb** - pot roast, mashed potatoes and green beans, for instance. Often converting a meal to a Fat Loss Plate is simply a matter of adjusting the portions of each component (American meals tend to be very **Fast Carb**-heavy) and tweaking the preparation just a touch.

Say your family loves spaghetti and meatballs. Just choose whole wheat pasta (or even pasta made with semolina or durum wheat), and some lower fat ingredients in your favorite meatball recipe (we've included a great recipe that is low in fat and high in flavor, or adapt your own recipe), then increase the ratio of meatballs to pasta following the guidelines of the Fat Loss Plate and... Voila! *You can lose weight eating spaghetti and meatballs*.

And if you want dessert but you've already had a **Fast Carb** with dinner, just wait 2 hours and enjoy a slice of Mom's Apple Pie (*Classic Comfort Food Recipe Cards*) with your coffee.

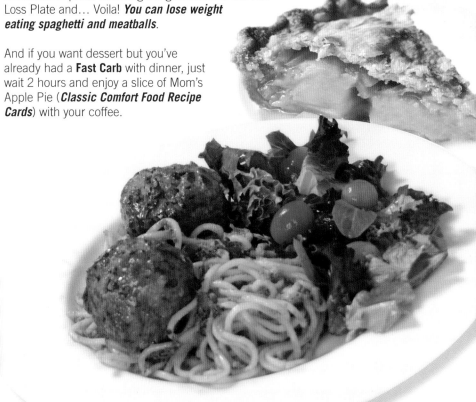

DAY 11

LORI B's FAVORITE
FAT LOSS MEAL

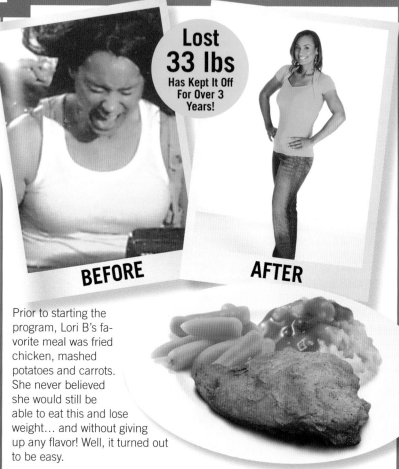

Lost 33 lbs
Has Kept It Off For Over 3 Years!

BEFORE

AFTER

Prior to starting the program, Lori B's favorite meal was fried chicken, mashed potatoes and carrots. She never believed she would still be able to eat this and lose weight… and without giving up any flavor! Well, it turned out to be easy.

The fried chicken was obviously the **Protein**. Chicken breast is already pretty lean, but instead of deep-frying in harmful Trans Fats, she experienced "oven-frying" with Southern "Oven Fried" Chicken in the ***Classic Comfort Food Recipe Cards*** to keep her metabolism humming away. The mashed potatoes are the **Fast Carb**. She chose to try the Mouthwatering Mashed Potatoes on page 111 in ***The Love to Eat Cookbook***, and as she says, her mouth really watered. Finally, for her **Slow Carb** she tried our recipe for Maple-Glazed Carrots in the ***Million Meals Menu Planner***. Then she served it all up in the right portion sizes for a Fat Loss Plate and her whole family loved it! She lost weight and her husband and kids had a healthier meal… and they never knew the difference.

DO THIS TODAY

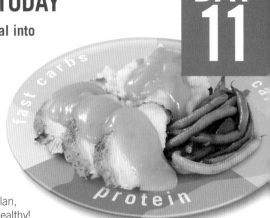

1 **Turn Your Family's Favorite Meal into a Fat Loss Plate**

Today, cook a meal that you and your family love but that you haven't had since you started the program. If you don't have a family favorite recipe pick one from the *The Love to Eat Cookbook* or the *Classic Comfort Food Recipe Cards* that sounds good and give it a try. You don't even have to tell your family it's healthier. That's one of the truly great things about the **Food Lovers Fat Loss System** – on this plan, everyone in your family gets lean and healthy!

2 **Remember:**

You are more than half way through the *21 Day Metabolism Makeover* and for the remaining week and a half you are doing EVERYTHING you can to accelerate your metabolism:

- All of your meals are Fat Loss Plates; all your snacks are Accelerator Snacks
- You are eating a meal or snack every 2 to 3 hours
- You are eating breakfast within 30 to 60 minutes of waking
- You are drinking at least one extra 8-ounce glass of water a day and avoiding alcohol
- You are eating healthier breads, sweets and fats and cutting back on sodium
- You are doing 12 minutes of exercise every other day
- **You are loving what you eat!**

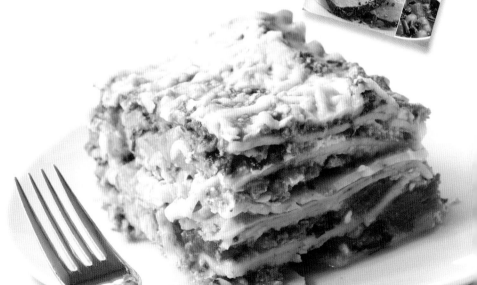

DAY 11

TURN YOUR FAMILY'S FAVORITE MEAL
INTO A FAT LOSS PLATE

Serve your family a Fat Loss Meal that they love which you haven't yet had on the program. Use the tips in *The Love to Eat Cookbook* to conver your family's favorite meal into a Fat Loss Plate or try something new from the cookbook or *Classic Comfort Food Recipes Cards*.

✓ TO DO'S
(check when done)

- [ ] Listen to the **Day 11** Audio Program
- [ ] Turn your family's favorite meal into a Fat Loss Plate
- [ ] Eat Fat Loss Meals and Accelerator Snacks every 2 to 3 hours
- [ ] Take my nutritional supplements
- [ ] Get 7 to 8 hours of sleep
- [ ] Choose only healthy breads, sweets and fats. Cut back on sodium.
- [ ] Drink more water and avoid alcohol
- [ ] _____
- [ ] _____
- [ ] _____
- [ ] _____

TODAY'S CALLS

_____
_____
_____
_____
_____
_____
_____
_____

TODAY'S SCHEDULE

B-FAST / SNACK: Time   **Mins. Since Waking Up:** Time
I ate/drank:

EAT!

7:00 am

8:00 am

9:00 am

B-FAST / SNACK: Time   **Hours Since Breakfast:** Time
I ate/drank:

EAT!

10:00 am

11:00 am

12:00 pm

LUNCH / SNACK: Time   **Hours Since Snack:** Time
I ate/drank:

EAT!

1:00 pm

2:00 pm

SNACK: Time   **Hours Since Lunch:** Time
I ate/drank:

EAT!

EXERCISE   ☐ YES   ☐ NO   TIME [   ]

What/how much?
_____
_____

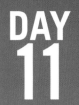

HAVING TROUBLE?

If you think you're not losing weight as fast as you should be or that you've hit a plateau, check out the **Fat Loss Trouble-shooter** on page 34 of the *Rapid Results Success Journal* for a step-by-step guide for getting back on track today!

TODAY'S SCHEDULE

3:00 pm

4:00 pm

5:00 pm

DINNER: Time   **Hours Since Snack:** Time

ate/drank:

EAT!

6:00 pm

7:00 pm

8:00 pm

SNACK: Time   **Hours Since Dinner:** Time

ate/drank:

EAT!

9:00 pm

10:00 pm

SNACK: Time   **Hours Since Snack:** Time

ate/drank:

EAT!

11:00 pm

Time I Went to Bed: Time

WHICH WOULD YOU RATHER HAVE?

A chicken breast deep-fried in harmful Trans Fats for
600 calories...

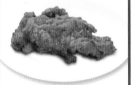

OR

a scrumptious, equally-juicy chicken breast oven-fried with zero Trans Fats and only
170 calories?

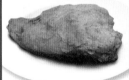

Turn to pages 31 to 40 of *The Love to Eat Cookbook* now to learn how you can turn your family's favorite meals into Fat Loss Plates that keep your body in "Fat Burning Mode!"

NOTES

For each 8 oz. glass of water consumed, CIRCLE A NUMBER ➜ 1 2 3 4 5 6 7 8 9 10 11 12

How many hours did you sleep last night? _____

Supplements I took today? _____

Now that you've discovered how delicious losing weight can be, it's time to learn how to increase your fat burning potential so you can **burn more calories all day long... even while you sleep!**

DAY: 12
DO 12 MINUTES
OF
RESISTANCE TRAINING

Today, instead of doing 12 Minutes of Fat Burning Cardio you are going to do 12 Minutes of Lean Muscle Building Resistance Exercise. You can use machines or weights at the gym, do some calisthenics at home or simply pop in your *12 Minute Muscle Maker* video and follow along. This specially-designed video is the fastest and easiest way to work your whole body and build the lean muscle tissue that will help you burn more calories all day long - all in just 12 minutes. Then, from now on, alternate your Fat Burning and Resistance workouts every other day.

What is
Resistance Exercise?

Simply put, Resistance Exercise is any movement where your body exerts a force against some kind of resistance (i.e., pushing, squeezing, etc.). This resistance can come from weights – dumbbells, barbells or any other heavy object. It can be provided by machines in the gym – using weight stacks, rubber bands or springs – or it can come from your own body weight as is the case with push-ups, sit-ups, squats, etc. Resistance Exercise is used to develop the strength and size of skeletal muscles.

Burn More Calories with Resistance Training

The biggest reason to do resistance training is to increase your lean muscle tissue. Lean muscle is responsible for burning 98% of the fat we want to get rid of… so the more lean muscle tissue you build, the more fat you'll burn.

And it gets even better… When you perform resistance training you give your metabolism a calorie-burning boost. Simply put, not only do you burn calories during your resistance training session – you boost your metabolism and burn more calories for the rest of the day.

What Else Do I Get From Resistance Training?

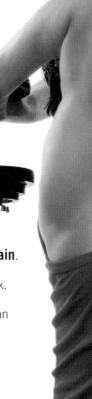

- **Stronger muscles, which in turn means stronger bones**, thus reducing the risk of osteoporosis and fractures.

- **An improvement in blood cholesterol levels**. Lifting weights may also help control blood pressure and blood sugar.

- **Less risk of injury during other activities**. It can help correct muscle weakness and imbalances and improve joint instability.

- **Improved self-esteem and self-confidence**. Added muscle and bone strength will benefit you in your daily activities, including other exercises and sports.

- **Reduced arthritis pain and lower-back pain**.

- **MORE fat loss** and less risk of gaining it back.

- **Lean muscle just <u>LOOKS</u> better!** A firm, lean physique is almost universally thought of as highly attractive.

Making It Happen!

You can do a resistance workout virtually anywhere with little or no equipment. The quickest and easiest way to do it is to simply pop in your *12 Minute Muscle Maker* video and follow along. All you need are some dumbbells or, if you don't have those, you can start with some objects from the pantry or fridge - some soup cans or water bottles - anything that has weight will provide resistance.

If you prefer, you can also go to the gym or health club. Check out our website for information about maximizing your workout in the gym. If you choose to do your workout in the gym or health club, you should start with what's called a **circuit** – where, for example, you do 1 to 3 sets of 8 to 15 repetitions on each of the different machines – one for each muscle group. (A "repetition" is one performance of a muscle move such as one bicep curl; a "set" is a collection of "reps" done without interruption.) This ensures that all your muscle groups get a workout.

The one key to resistance is to always make sure that you are increasing intensity from one workout to the next. Otherwise, as your body gets stronger, it will adapt to the exercises **quickly** and you'll get less benefit from the same workout. The simplest way to avoid this is to increase the amount of resistance slightly. If you are using 50 pounds or less for your resistance, increase the weight by 10%. If you are using 50 pounds or more for your resistance, increase the weight by 5%. If you're not able to increase the resistance weight, you can increase the number of sets you do, but do not exceed 4 sets. This ensures that you are always getting the most from your workout.

Doing any kind of exercise can quickly deplete the available sugar (your body's source of energy) in your bloodstream and lean muscle tissue. So it is important that you eat before AND after a resistance workout.

• If You Workout First-thing in the Morning...
Be sure to eat either a snack or Fat Loss Breakfast prior to your workout. This is particularly important for resistance workouts. Then wait at least 30 to 60 minutes for the food to digest so it won't cause discomfort when exercising.

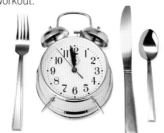

• Eat Within One Hour After Working Out...
Resistance exercise will deplete your body's energy supplies very quickly, so to avoid a drop in sugar levels that could cause uncontrollable cravings or an insulin surge, regardless of your eating schedule so far, **eat a Fat Loss Meal within one hour of working out. This is imperative, but if you can't quite eat a full Fat Loss Meal, at least eat a Fat Loss Snack within one hour of working out. And then make sure you get back on-schedule by eating a full Fat Loss Meal 2 to 3 hours after that snack.**

From beginning to end, this is roughly a 2-hour interval, which puts you right on-schedule with your **Food Lovers** eating plan. As you can see, it's important to coordinate your exercising and eating schedules so that they work together to keep you consistently in "Fat Burning Mode."

DO THIS TODAY

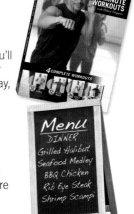

1 ### Do 12 Minutes of Resistance Training
Today, increase your fat burning potential by doing 12 minutes of Resistance Training. Then going forward, you'll exercise for 12 minutes every other day, alternating your cardio and your resistance training. Example: on Monday, do cardio; on Wednesday, do resistance; on Friday do cardio again, and so on.

2 ### Make a Dinner Reservation for Tomorrow
Tomorrow you are going to learn how to order a Fat Loss Plate at your favorite restaurant. So decide where you are going to go and, if needed, make a reservation.

Menu
DINNER
Grilled Halibut
Seafood Medley
BBQ Chicken
Rib Eye Steak
Shrimp Scampi

DAY 12

DO 12 MINUTES OF RESISTANCE TRAINGING

In place of your cardio workout, do 12 Minutes of Resistance Training today. Hit the gym or simply pop in your *12 Minute Muscle Maker DVD* and start to build the lean, attractive muscle tissue that will have you burning more calories all day long.

✓ TO DO'S
(check when done)

- ☐ Listen to the **Day 12** Audio Program
- ☐ Do 12 minutes of Resistance Training
- ☐ Eat Fat Loss Meals and Accelerator Snacks every 2 to 3 hours
- ☐ Take my nutritional supplements
- ☐ Get 7 to 8 hours of sleep
- ☐ Choose only healthy breads, sweets and fats. Cut back on sodium.
- ☐ Drink more water and avoid alcohol
- ☐ Pick a restaurant for tomorrow
- ☐ _____
- ☐ _____
- ☐ _____
- ☐ _____

TODAY'S CALLS

_____
_____
_____
_____
_____
_____

TODAY'S SCHEDULE

B-FAST / SNACK: Time   **Mins. Since Waking Up:** Time

I ate/drank:

EAT! protein

7:00 am

8:00 am

9:00 am

B-FAST / SNACK: Time   **Hours Since Breakfast:** Time

I ate/drank:

EAT! protein

10:00 am

11:00 am

12:00 pm

LUNCH / SNACK: Time   **Hours Since Snack:** Time

I ate/drank:

EAT! protein

1:00 pm

2:00 pm

SNACK: Time   **Hours Since Lunch:** Time

I ate/drank:

EAT! protein

EXERCISE ☐ YES ☐ NO   TIME

What/how much?

_____
_____

DID YOU KNOW...

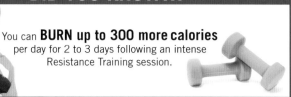

You can **BURN up to 300 more calories** per day for 2 to 3 days following an intense Resistance Training session.

TODAY'S SCHEDULE

3:00 pm _____

4:00 pm _____

5:00 pm _____

DINNER: Time   **Hours Since Snack:** Time

te/drank:

EAT! _____

6:00 pm _____

7:00 pm _____

8:00 pm _____

SNACK: Time   **Hours Since Dinner:** Time

te/drank:

EAT! _____

9:00 pm _____

0:00 pm _____

SNACK: Time   **Hours Since Snack:** Time

te/drank:

EAT! _____

1:00 pm _____

Time I Went to Bed: Time

RESISTANCE EXERCISE MYTHS

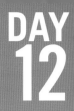

I'm Too Old for Resistance Training. FALSE! Age does not matter when it comes to Resistance Training. As a matter of fact, if you're over 50, Resistance Training can be your best friend. Plus the older and more out of shape you are the faster and more dramatically you will benefit from Resistance Training.

Resistance will Make Women Look Like a Body Builder. FALSE! Women simply do not have enough testosterone to cause muscles to grow big and bulky. What you will get are shapely, beautiful arms, legs and shoulders (to name a few) and an increase in fat burning potential.

It Takes a Long Time. FALSE! Unlike cardio, resistance exercise is very quick. If you think about it, doing one set of an exercise takes about thirty seconds. Your _12 Minute Muscle Maker DVD_ works every single muscle group in your body in only 12 minutes.

NOTES

For each 8 oz. glass of water consumed, **CIRCLE A NUMBER** ➜ 1   2   3   4   5   6   7   8   9   10   11   12

ow many hours did you sleep last night? _____

upplements I took today? _____

For the last week you've been eating in a way that guarantees you'll lose weight fast. Today you're going to hone the skills that will make sure you can keep it off for the rest of your life.

DAY 13: ORDER
A FAT LOSS PLATE
AT YOUR FAVORITE RESTAURANT

Today you are going to prove to yourself that you really can eat in a way that will cause you to lose weight not just during the first 21 days but for the rest of your life and… anywhere you go. First, **read over the *Eating Out Advisor*, then grab your spouse, or round up the kids, and head out to your favorite restaurant.** It can be breakfast, lunch or dinner. **Just follow the guidelines of the Food Lovers program and order a Fat Loss Meal that you love**.

A Plan That Fits Your Lifestyle

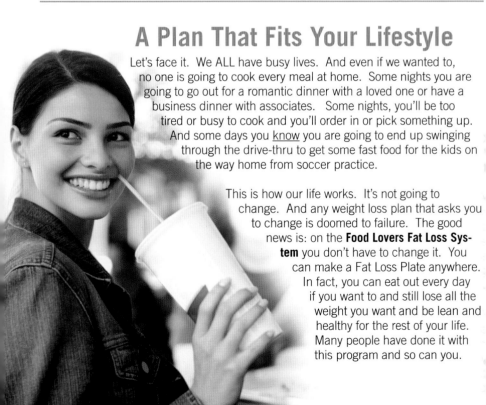

Let's face it. We ALL have busy lives. And even if we wanted to, no one is going to cook every meal at home. Some nights you are going to go out for a romantic dinner with a loved one or have a business dinner with associates. Some nights, you'll be too tired or busy to cook and you'll order in or pick something up. And some days you <u>know</u> you are going to end up swinging through the drive-thru to get some fast food for the kids on the way home from soccer practice.

This is how our life works. It's not going to change. And any weight loss plan that asks you to change is doomed to failure. The good news is: on the **Food Lovers Fat Loss System** you don't have to change it. You can make a Fat Loss Plate anywhere. In fact, you can eat out every day if you want to and still lose all the weight you want and be lean and healthy for the rest of your life. Many people have done it with this program and so can you.

Ordering Out at Restaurants

Ordering a meal that will cause you to lose weight at a restaurant isn't really any more difficult than doing it at home – which is to say, not difficult at all. The two biggest challenges with trying to eat in a way that will make you lean and healthy at restaurants are 1) the Portion sizes are often too large (particularly the portion of **Fast Carbs**), and 2) you don't know how they prepared the food – how much hidden fat and other metabolism-slowing ingredients were used in the cooking. Still, once you know what you are doing, getting a meal guaranteed to switch your body into "Fat Burning Mode" and cause you to lose weight is easy.

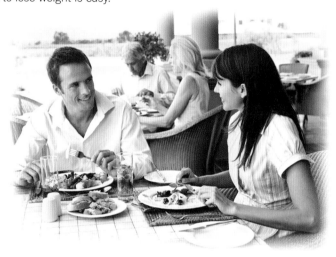

Making a Fat Loss Plate at Your Favorite Restaurant

Constructing a Fat Loss Plate at a restaurant is pretty much the same as doing it at home. You start by asking yourself the two basic questions: "What is my **Protein** going to be?" and then "What are my **Fast and Slow Carbs** going to be?"

All restaurants have some sort of **Protein**, and obviously, the leaner the better. Fish, chicken breast, and lean steak are all great choices and nearly every restaurant offers one or all of these. **Fast Carbs** are even easier. Baked potato, rice, whole grain bread in a sandwich, pasta, and (after your *21 day Metabolism Makeover* – even a glass of wine) are all great **Fast Carbs**. And then you just round it out with a **Slow Carb** – a fibrous veggie liked steamed broccoli, spinach or asparagus, a vegetable soup or a green salad all work. It's that simple.

And even if you can't find a meal with the right ratios on the menu, restaurants will almost always mix and match sides. So if the entrée you are looking for contains too many **Fast Carbs**, have them substitute some **Slow Carb** veggies for one of them. Often you can essentially build your own meal. Start with a **Protein** then scan the menu for the **Slow** and **Fast Carbs** that sound best to you. Just be friendly and specific when placing your order and they'll almost always be happy to accommodate you.

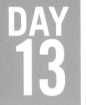

Portion Sizes

This is where it gets a bit tricky. Portions in restaurants have gotten bigger and bigger over the past decade, and it is no coincidence that this fact corresponds with increasing levels of obesity in this country. Reference the portion chart in *How to Make a Fat Loss Plate*, then, as soon as your meal comes, identify the right size portion of each food and separate it from the rest. Take the rest home or back to the office. Have the leftovers for your snack a few hours later. With the portion sizes in some restaurants, you may actually end up with several full meals for the price of one!

The "Enemies of Fat Loss"

The other things to watch out for are ingredients with high amounts of fat, refined sugars and flours, and other "Enemies of Fat Loss." At home you know what goes in your food; at a restaurant you'd be amazed at the vast amounts of calories they can pack into a few tablespoons of salad dressing or in the little bit of sauce drizzled over your fish.

Get What You Want

Fortunately, as Americans have gotten more health conscious, restaurants have gotten much more accommodating of special requests. The best way to stay in control is to have them bring the sauces and dressings on the side. That way YOU get to choose how much of these ingredients you want to add to your food. And, just like at home where you choose to leave out the biggest "enemies of fat loss" in the preparation of your food when you can't taste them, at a restaurant you can make the same requests – "Can you please grill that without oil or butter?" "Just steam the veggies please and I'll add any oil or butter myself here at the table if I want it."

Don't be afraid to ask for food to be prepared the way you want. Again, you are the customer, you are paying and most restaurants will be happy to accommodate you. Just be specific.

Enjoy Your Meal

Perhaps the most important thing to remember when eating out on the **Food Lovers** program is: **enjoy your meal**. Order what you want. If you only order grilled fish and steamed veggies every time you go out, you'll start to take the joy out of eating. And enjoying what you eat is one of the cornerstones of this program. It's what makes it work for the long term. So just do the best you can. As long as you stick to the right combinations and portion sizes for a Fat Loss Plate, you'll never be too far off.

By ordering a Fat Loss Plate at your favorite restaurant, you will gain the wisdom, knowledge, and skill to dine out without fear, apprehension or discomfort.

DO THIS TODAY

1 **Order a Fat Loss Meal at Your Favorite Restaurant**
Read over the **Eating Out Advisor**, then grab your friends and family and head out to your favorite restaurant. Prove to yourself that you can eat in a way that will make you lean and healthy anywhere – without giving up the food you love – by ordering a Fat Loss Meal at your favorite eating establishment.

2 **Review Your Planner Pages UP to This Point**
As of tomorrow, you will have been on the **21 Day Metabolism Makeover** for two weeks. Take a look back over your Planner Pages so far. Have you been eating every 2 to 3 hours? Keeping to the combination and pro-portions of the Fat Loss Plate? Choosing only the healthiest breads and sweets? Doing your 12 minute fat burning and resistance exercises? Start to look for connections between how you ate and exercised and how you felt, how your clothes are fitting. Start to associate healthy eating and exercise with the results you are getting.

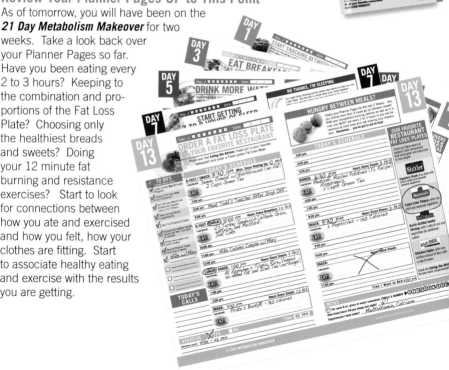

DAY 13

ORDER A FAT LOSS PLATE AT YOUR FAVORITE RESTAURANT

Read over the *Eating Out Advisor*, head out to your favorite restaurant and order a **Food Lovers Fat Loss Meal**.

✓ TO DO'S
(check when done)

- [ ] Listen to the **Day 13** Audio Program
- [ ] Order a Fat Loss Meal at a restaurant
- [ ] Eat Fat Loss Meals and Accelerator Snacks every 2 to 3 hours
- [ ] Take my nutritional supplements
- [ ] Get 7 to 8 hours of sleep
- [ ] Choose only healthy breads, sweets and fats. Cut back on sodium.
- [ ] Drink more water and avoid alcohol
- [ ] Review Planner Pages from last 2 weeks
- [ ] _____
- [ ] _____
- [ ] _____
- [ ] _____

TODAY'S CALLS

_____
_____
_____
_____
_____

TODAY'S SCHEDULE

B-FAST / SNACK: Time   **Mins. Since Waking Up:** Time

I ate/drank:

EAT! Protein

7:00 am

8:00 am

9:00 am

B-FAST / SNACK: Time   **Hours Since Breakfast:** Time

I ate/drank:

EAT! Protein

10:00 am

11:00 am

12:00 pm

LUNCH / SNACK: Time   **Hours Since Snack:** Time

I ate/drank:

EAT! Protein

1:00 pm

2:00 pm

SNACK: Time   **Hours Since Lunch:** Time

I ate/drank:

EAT! Protein

EXERCISE ☐ YES ☐ NO   **TIME** _____

What/how much?

_____
_____

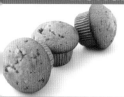

HUNGRY BETWEEN MEALS?

Check your Planner Pages for the last 2 Weeks. Are you letting more than 3 hours go by between meals? With your metabolism burning calories as fast as it is now, you MUST eat every 2 to 3 hours or you will be ravenous at meal time and risk slowing your metabolism. **Remember... you've got to eat to lose!**

TODAY'S SCHEDULE

3:00 pm

4:00 pm

5:00 pm

DINNER: Time   **Hours Since Snack:** Time

ate/drank:

EAT!

6:00 pm

7:00 pm

8:00 pm

SNACK: Time   **Hours Since Dinner:** Time

ate/drank:

EAT!

9:00 pm

10:00 pm

SNACK: Time   **Hours Since Snack:** Time

ate/drank:

EAT!

11:00 pm

Time I Went to Bed: Time

OUR FAVORITE RESTAURANT FAT LOSS PLATES

Check out these meals at national chain restaurants that **taste great and cause you to lose weight:**

Sizzler

Signature Steak: 8 oz steak with baked potato and steamed seasonal vegetables.

Applebee's
Neighborhood Grill & Bar

Cajun Lime Tilapia: with rice pilaf and seasonal vegetables

Red Lobster

Garlic-Grilled Jumbo Shrimp: with a side of rice and vegetables (no additional butter)

BAJA FRESH
MEXICAN · GRILL

Chicken Fajita: with corn tortillas instead of flour with a side of beans

Check the *Eating Out Advisor* for even more recommendations.

NOTES

For each 8 oz. glass of water consumed, **CIRCLE A NUMBER** ➜ 1 2 3 4 5 6 7 8 9 10 11 12

How many hours did you sleep last night? _____

Supplements I took today? _____

One of the primary reasons people lose motivation and get off track of their goal to win at weight loss, is a lack of support. So today you're going to make sure you **have all the support you need to get the body you've always dreamed of.**

DAY 14:
LOG ON TO THE WEBSITE AND FIND A FOOD LOVERS FAT LOSS BUDDY

Log on to our website at **chat.MyFoodLovers.com** and find yourself a **Food Lovers Fat Loss Buddy**. Check out all the **Food Lovers Fat Loss Forums**, read over the messages, and find someone you "connect" with someone who shares your interests and your concerns, or who lives near you or has a similar lifestyle or weight loss goal. Then send her/him an Instant Message (IM) . Introduce yourself and let them know what you are looking for someone who will commit to be your **Food Lovers Fat Loss Buddy**. Make arrangements to stay in touch regularly (on the Forums, by e-mail or IM) to keep each other motivated, share recipes and snack ideas and support one another whenever obstacles present themselves. It may seem a small thing, but it can make a HUGE difference.

We're Here to Help

Psychologists and weight-watching organizations have learned that the support of two or more people can not only boost motivation, but increase your likelihood of seeing your weight loss goals through. You are probably aware of entire weight loss programs that are virtually nothing more than support and motivation from peers at scheduled weekly meetings. And that's because it works. In fact, in Robert Ferguson's years of research and coaching thousands of people to win at weight loss, he knows as well as anyone that being a part of a group or team with a common goal is one of the surest methods for guaranteeing your success!

The good news is, research shows that you don't need to attend weekly meetings or pay weekly fees to enjoy the motivational benefits offered by these sorts of programs. You can get the same kind of support that can increase your weight loss and make it easier to keep it off in the comfort and privacy of your own home.

Food Lovers Online

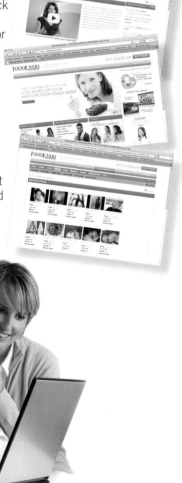

We are committed to giving you all the support you need all the way through your journey until you reach your goals and beyond. And our website is the best place to start.

Today, set aside a minimum of 30 minutes to log onto the website and check out all it has to offer. Start with our extensive Chat Forums. These were custom-designed to allow anyone to get all the help and resources they need to succeed 24 hours a day. You'll find people from all over the country just like you – who can help you in any way you might need.

- **Need some new recipes?** Check out the Recipe Forums where Food Lovers from all over the country have posted recipes that they love and that they have used to lose weight.
- **Getting bored of your snacks?** Check out the Snack Forums to find out what others are eating, where to buy the tastiest snacks, and get tasty recipes for satisfying your sweet tooth.
- **Got a LOT of weight to lose?** We've got weight-based Forums where you can get tips and tricks from people who started where you are now – no matter how much weight you have to lose. Find out how they did it and let them keep you motivated until you reach your goal.
- **Want to find someone in your area who's on the program?** Search the Forums by city, state or zip code to create a local network of **Food Lovers**. Get together in person to help keep each other excited and motivated.
- **Need a Pep Talk in the middle of the night?** There's always someone on the Forums -- no matter what time of day -- ready to lend an ear and help you past whatever obstacle you may face.

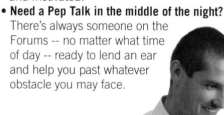

That's Just the Beginning

We are committed to providing you all the resources you need to achieve the results you want. So check back often for our growing list of online resources:

- More Great Tasting Fat Loss Recipes
- Snack Ideas, Restaurant Recommendations, etc.
- Support from Our Specially-Trained Fat Loss Specialists
- And much, much more…

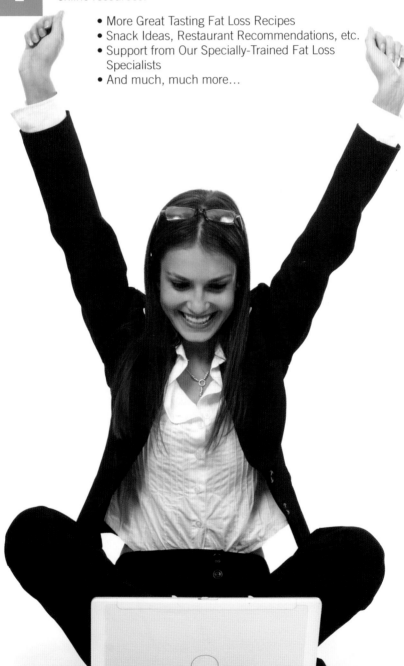

DO THIS TODAY

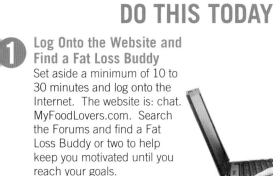

1 **Log Onto the Website and Find a Fat Loss Buddy**
Set aside a minimum of 10 to 30 minutes and log onto the Internet. The website is: chat.MyFoodLovers.com. Search the Forums and find a Fat Loss Buddy or two to help keep you motivated until you reach your goals.

2 **Reward Yourself**
Congratulations! You've finished your second week on the program and are already two-thirds of the way through your *21 Day Metabolism Makeover*. Your body is now burning fat as fast as possible, and over the next week, you will see some amazing results. It's time to give yourself another reward for the great work you did last week. Turn to page 29 of your *Rapid Results Success Journal* and give yourself the reward you promised yourself today. You've already set the reward for next week, for when you complete the first phase of the program, so all you've got to do today is kick back and enjoy your reward... and your success -- you deserve it!

3 **Get Ready for Tomorrow**
Tomorrow you are going to do a FUN Fat Burning Activity. You'll see that a workout doesn't actually have to be "work" to give you great results. Read over the day, decide what "fun" activity you'd like to use to accelerate your fat burning, and make sure to schedule it.

MAKE PERFECTION YOUR GOAL

Never wait even one minute beyond 3 hours to eat; Choose only the healthiest breads and sweets; Get 7 to 8 hours of sleep per night.

DAY 14

Day: ✓ S M T W TH F S   **Date:** ___ / ___ / ___

LOG ON TO THE WEBSITE
AND FIND A FOOD LOVERS FAT LOSS BUDDY

Go to your computer, log onto www.MyFoodLovers.com and spen
time exploring the resources. Find a Fat Loss Buddy and arrang
to communicate regularly until you both reach your fat loss goal

✓ TO DO'S
(check when done)

☐ Listen to the **Day 14** Audio Program

☐ Log onto the website and find a Fat Loss Buddy

☐ Reward yourself and set a new weekly goal

☐ Do 12 minutes of Fat Burning Cardio

☐ Eat Fat Loss Meals and Accelerator Snacks every 2 to 3 hours

☐ Take my nutritional supplements

☐ Get 7 to 8 hours of sleep

☐ Choose only healthy breads, sweets and fats. Cut back on sodium.

☐ Drink more water and avoid alcohol

☐ Plan tomorrow's "fun" fat burning activity

☐ _____

☐ _____

☐ _____

☐ _____

TODAY'S CALLS

_____

_____

_____

_____

TODAY'S SCHEDULE

B-FAST / SNACK: Time   **Mins. Since Waking Up:** Time

I ate/drank:

EAT! Protein

7:00 am

8:00 am

9:00 am

B-FAST / SNACK: Time   **Hours Since Breakfast:** Time

I ate/drank:

EAT! Protein

10:00 am

11:00 am

12:00 pm

LUNCH / SNACK: Time   **Hours Since Snack:** Time

I ate/drank:

EAT! Protein

1:00 pm

2:00 pm

SNACK: Time   **Hours Since Lunch:** Time

I ate/drank:

EAT! Protein

EXERCISE   ☐ YES   ☐ NO   **TIME** [_____]

What/how much?

_____

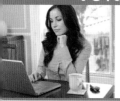

75% ARE JUST LIKE YOU

Today, 3 out of 4 Americans own a computer – that's 75% of the population – and that means 75% of **Food Lovers** like yourself are probably out looking for a Fat Loss Buddy to keep them motivated just like you are. Take the time to log on NOW at chat.MyFoodLovers.com!

TODAY'S SCHEDULE

3:00 pm _____

4:00 pm _____

5:00 pm _____

DINNER: Time   **Hours Since Snack:** Time

te/drank: _____

EAT! _____

6:00 pm _____

7:00 pm _____

8:00 pm _____

SNACK: Time   **Hours Since Dinner:** Time

te/drank: _____

EAT! _____

9:00 pm _____

10:00 pm _____

SNACK: Time   **Hours Since Snack:** Time

e/drank: _____

EAT! _____

11:00 pm _____

Time I Went to Bed: Time

ULTIMATE FAT LOSS BUDDIES

Kim L.
Lost
63 lbs

BEFORE   AFTER

Kim L. struggled with weight her entire life. When she started The Food Lovers plan, she found her Fat Loss Buddy in her very own home – her son, Ethan.

Ethan L.
Lost
100 lbs

BEFORE   AFTER

Ethan L., at just 16 years old, had been struggling with his weight for most of his relatively short life too. Together, their support, love, and care have resulted in nearly 170 pounds of total fat loss!

NOTES

For each 8 oz. glass of water consumed, **CIRCLE A NUMBER** ➜ 1 2 3 4 5 6 7 8 9 10 11 12

w many hours did you sleep last night? _____

pplements I took today? _____

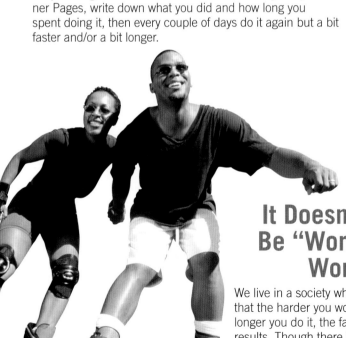

Not everybody loves to work out. But everybody loves to do *something* that involves some physical activity. Today we're going to teach you how to **maximize fat burning while doing something "fun."**

DAY 15:
DO A "FUN"
FAT BURNING
ACTIVITY

Follow the directions here and do a fun physical activity which you like – golf, tennis, hiking, shooting hoops with the kids, window shopping at the mall will even work – as long as you keep moving for at least 30 minutes continuously. In your Planner Pages, write down what you did and how long you spent doing it, then every couple of days do it again but a bit faster and/or a bit longer.

It Doesn't Have to Be "Work" to Be a Workout!

We live in a society where most people believe that the harder you work at exercise and the longer you do it, the faster you're going to see results. Though there is some truth to this, it's not the most practical approach, and burning fat can be achieved in far easier ways.

Anytime you are up and moving around, you are burning calories. If you are moving fast enough to keep your heart elevated to a point where you're not out of breath but are beginning to perspire, you are burning A LOT OF CALORIES.

Turning the activities you love into activities that also burn fat is not as hard as you might think. You can do it easily with intense activities like tennis, racquetball or basketball, but it can also be accomplished with something as simple as playing tag with the kids in the back yard. The main thing you need to do to make sure that you are burning fat is keep moving continuously for a period of time – shoot for 30 minutes to start.

Make ANY Activity a Fat Burning Activity

Make a list of all the physical activities that you like to do and then find a way to tweak them so you are moving continuously. If you choose to play golf, for instance, instead of getting a cart and driving from hole to hole – walk, maybe even carry your clubs. If you like to window shop, start by power walking up and down the street for half an hour, deciding which shops you want to check out, before you actually head into the stores.

Track It, Then AMP It Up

As we've said before, the best way to maximize results is by constantly increasing some aspect of your workout -- either intensity or duration. So keep track of what you do, then next time you do it, try to do it faster or longer. For instance, keep track of how long it takes you to play 9 or 18 holes, then on your way out, schedule another tee time several days later and see if you can play the same amount of holes in a faster amount of time. If you kick the soccer ball with the kids for a half hour today, tomorrow go for 45 minutes -- and run a bit harder. Every time you do a "fun" fat burning activity, record the details in your Planner Pages and next time… amp it up!

THE THREE PHASES OF A
WORKOUT

Ideally, every fat burning activity has three phases:
❶ Warm-Up   ❷ Workout   ❸ Cool-Down

Try to incorporate all three phases into your "fun" workout. If you choose to play tennis, start easy, just volleying the ball back and forth, then note when you really start to "play" -- that's your workout.   Finally, note when you stop playing and do another few minutes of cool down – maybe stroll around the park.   If you choose to go walking with a friend, approach it the same way.   During the first few minutes, walk a bit more slowly then note the time and crank it up for your "workout."   When you're done, spend another few minutes cooling down. Make sure to keep track of time spent warming up and cooling down as well as your actual "workout" in your Planner Pages.

By making sure every workout also includes good warm-up and cool-down segments, you'll do two things: (1) help prevent injuries and (2) decrease the amount of time your muscles need to recover, so try to make sure that all your work-outs include all of the three phases.

Make TIME for FUN

BEWARE! For some odd reason, when it comes to trying to carve out some time to have some fun, something always seems to come up and get in the way of you taking time to enjoy yourself. On the other hand, when it's time for work, there always seems to be plenty of time to get it done. If you want to get lean, healthy and happy, **you need to give "having fun" the same priority you give to "work."**

Use this time to socialize. Get to know a co-worker better with a friendly game of racquetball. Spend some time with your brother or an old buddy on the golf course. Go walking with your neighbor. Just make sure that your activity doesn't *rely* on the other person for you to still do it. Always have a back-up activity you enjoy, so if your sister cancels the hike in the woods, you don't have to give up your fat burning.

DO THIS TODAY

1 **Do a "FUN" Fat Burning Activity**
Find a "fun" activity and do it in a way that has you moving continuously for 30 minutes or more today. Write down what you did and for how long in your Planner Pages then schedule more "fun" fat burning activities every few days – going a bit farther or faster each time you do it.

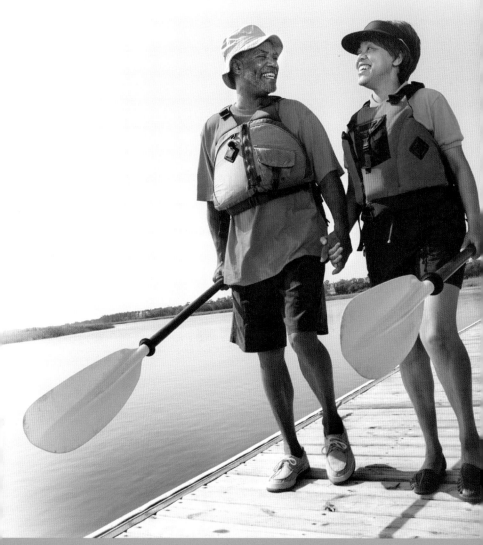

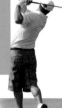

DAY 15

DO A "FUN"
FAT BURNING ACTIVITY

Choose some physical activity that you truly enjoy today -- anything from golf or tennis to playing with the kids, and find a way to do it in a way that keeps you moving continuously for 30 minutes or more. Record the details in your Planner Pages.

✓ TO DO'S
(check when done)

- ☐ Listen to the **Day 15** Audio Program
- ☐ Do a "fun" fat burning activity for 30 min today
- ☐ Eat Fat Loss Meals with Accelerator Snacks every 2 to 3 hours
- ☐ Take my nutritional supplements
- ☐ Get 7 to 8 hours of sleep
- ☐ Choose only healthy breads, sweets and fats. Cut back on sodium.
- ☐ Drink more water and avoid alcohol
- ☐ _____
- ☐ _____
- ☐ _____
- ☐ _____

TODAY'S CALLS

_____
_____
_____
_____
_____
_____
_____

TODAY'S SCHEDULE

B-FAST / SNACK: Time　　　　　　**Mins. Since Waking Up:** Time

I ate/drank:

EAT!

7:00 am

8:00 am

9:00 am

B-FAST / SNACK: Time　　　　　　**Hours Since Breakfast:** Time

I ate/drank:

EAT!

10:00 am

11:00 am

12:00 pm

LUNCH / SNACK: Time　　　　　　**Hours Since Snack:** Time

I ate/drank:

EAT!

1:00 pm

2:00 pm

SNACK: Time　　　　　　**Hours Since Lunch:** Time

I ate/drank:

EAT!

EXERCISE ☐ YES ☐ NO　　　　TIME [_____]

What/how much?

_____
_____

FAT LOSS TIP

Weight bearing exercises, where you are on your feet and carrying your own weight like walking, jogging, playing tennis, etc, will always burn more calories than non-weight bearing exercises like swimming or bicycling where the water or bicycle is holding you up.

TODAY'S SCHEDULE

3:00 pm

4:00 pm

5:00 pm

DINNER: Time   **Hours Since Snack:** Time

ate/drank:

EAT!

6:00 pm

7:00 pm

8:00 pm

SNACK: Time   **Hours Since Dinner:** Time

ate/drank:

EAT!

9:00 pm

10:00 pm

SNACK: Time   **Hours Since Snack:** Time

ate/drank:

EAT!

11:00 pm

Time I Went to Bed: Time

CALORIES BURNED IN COMMON ACTIVITIES

Gardening
(272 calories/hour)*

Ballroom Dancing
(306 calories/hour)*

Walking (3.0 MPH)
(224 calories per hour)*

Jogging
(789 calories/hour)*

Golf (Walking and Carrying Clubs)
(306 calories/hour)*

Tennis
(653 calories/hour)*

Water Skiing
(508 calories/hour)*

Hiking
(500 calories/hour)*

*based on a body weight of 150 lbs

NOTES

For each 8 oz. glass of water consumed, CIRCLE A NUMBER ➜ 1 2 3 4 5 6 7 8 9 10 11 12

How many hours did you sleep last night? _____

Supplements I took today? _____

DAY 16

This program is about making little changes that give you **huge** results, and today's activity is a great example of that. Starting today, you'll work out just a **little** bit longer, but by doing a new type of exercise you'll get **A LOT MORE** results.

DAY 16: EXERCISE FOR 24 MINUTES TODAY

Starting today, you are going to accelerate your results by upgrading your resistance exercise to 24 minutes. And, by doing the *24 Minute Burn & Tone DVD* workout, which uses the principles of "Circuit Training," you are actually going to get two workouts in one, so you'll get even faster results.

Two Workouts in One

The *24 Minute Burn & Tone DVD* employs what is known as "Circuit Training" which is widely acknowledged to be the most effective form of exercise you can do for fat loss. The main reason "Circuit Training" is so effective is that it combines both a resistance workout and a cardio workout in the same routine.

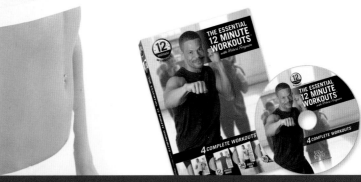

To get the benefits of fat burning cardio, you have to keep your heart rate elevated for an extended period of time. With "Circuit Training," you essentially do resistance exercises in a way that keeps your heart rate up – and in "Fat Burning Mode" – for your entire workout. Unlike conventional resistance exercises like weight-lifting where you rest between exercises, when you are "Circuit Training," you don't let your heart rate fall between exercises. You can do this in the gym or health club by going directly from machine to machine quickly, in a repeating circuit, working each body part without resting in between. This keeps your heart rate elevated – just like cardio workouts do – at the same time that you are building lean muscle tissue.

How Can I Work My Whole Body in Just 24 Minutes?

The other way to do "Circuit Training" is to alternate your resistance exercises with cardio exercises. This also keeps your heart rate way up for the entire workout, really amping up the benefits. This is also the secret of the ***24 Minute Burn and Tone DVD***, a fast, fun workout that has you going back and forth between simple resistance exercises and high-energy cardio movements. That's why it's called the ***24 Minute Burn and Tone DVD*** – the cardio moves keep you "burning" fat while the resistance exercises "tone" your problem areas, helping create a shapely, attractive figure and building the lean muscle that helps you burn more calories all day long.

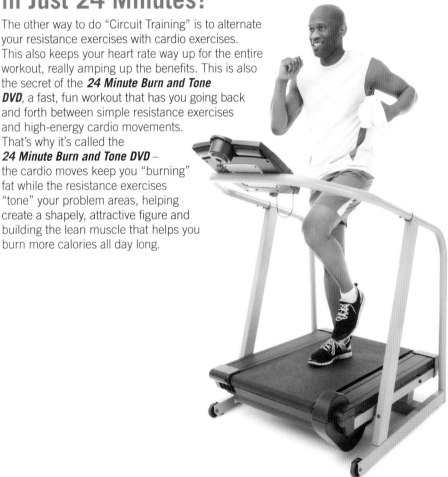

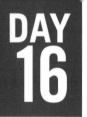

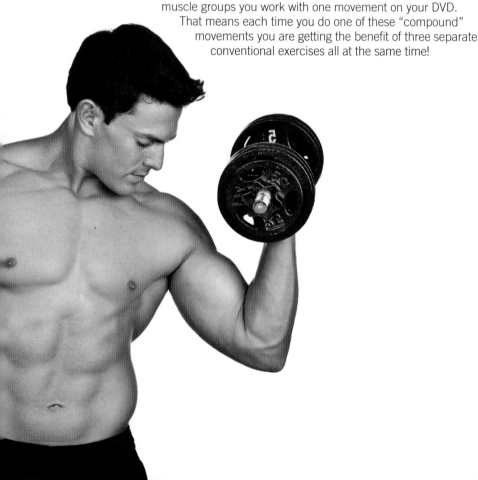

DAY 16

Compound Your Results

Not only does the *24 Minute Burn and Tone DVD* provide two workouts in one, but it can be much more efficient – in terms of time – than doing "Circuit Training" at the gym or health club. That is because when you work out on most weight machines in the gym or health club, you only work one muscle group at a time: curls work the biceps, arm extensions work your triceps, hip adduction works the inner thigh, and chest presses work the chest. But the resistance exercises featured on the DVD are different. They are known as "compound" movements because with each exercise you are actually working several different muscle groups at the same time. This means you can spend less time working out, but still enjoy all the body shaping benefits of more time-consuming fitness routines.

For instance, on the *24 Minute Burn and Tone DVD*, you'll be performing shoulder presses **at the same time** you are doing squats – which means you are working your shoulders with the presses AND your legs and your core muscles (abs, etc.) with the squats – all at the same time. In the gym you'd have to do shoulder presses, PLUS leg presses PLUS ab crunches – three separate movements – to work all the same muscle groups you work with one movement on your DVD. That means each time you do one of these "compound" movements you are getting the benefit of three separate conventional exercises all at the same time!

That's makes this kind of workout much more efficient. While it may take you an hour, or even two, to work every part of your body in the gym, with these videos, in just 24 minutes, you will literally work out every major muscle group in your body AND get a killer cardio workout at the same time.

DO THIS TODAY

1 **Exercise for 24 Minutes Today**
Starting today, replace your 12 minute resistance exercise with the ***24 Minute Burn and Tone DVD***. Alternately, you can do a full body "circuit" routine at the gym or health club, making sure to keep your heart rate consistently elevated while moving from exercise to exercise for at least 24 minutes.

2 **Get Ready for Tomorrow**
You are only going to eat meals and snacks that you love -- that are exciting and delicious. If anything even resembles "diet" food, it is off limits. So take a minute today and make a list of all your favorite dishes. If you haven't eaten them on the program yet, go through your materials (and log on to the website) and figure out how to make them in a way that will make your body burn fat.

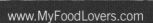

DAY 16

Day: ✓ S M T W TH F S Date: ___ / ___ / ___

EXERCISE FOR 24 MINUTES TODA

Do 24 minutes of resistance training today. Use the principles of "Circuit Training" by going from one exercise to the next without resting, or simply pop in the *24 Minute Burn and Tone DVD* and get two workouts in one -- in less than half an hour.

✓ TO DO'S
(check when done)

- ☐ Listen to the **Day 16** Audio Program
- ☐ Do 24 minutes of resistance exercise
- ☐ Eat Fat Loss Meals with Accelerator Snacks every 2 to 3 hours
- ☐ Take my nutritional supplements
- ☐ Get 7 to 8 hours of sleep
- ☐ Choose only healthy breads, sweets and fats. Cut back on sodium
- ☐ Drink more water and avoid alcohol
- ☐ _____
- ☐ _____
- ☐ _____
- ☐ _____

TODAY'S CALLS

_____
_____
_____
_____
_____
_____
_____

TODAY'S SCHEDULE

B-FAST / SNACK: Time   **Mins. Since Waking Up:** Time

I ate/drank:

EAT! Protein

7:00 am

8:00 am

9:00 am

B-FAST / SNACK: Time   **Hours Since Breakfast:** Time

I ate/drank:

EAT! Protein

10:00 am

11:00 am

12:00 pm

LUNCH / SNACK: Time   **Hours Since Snack:** Time

I ate/drank:

EAT! Protein

1:00 pm

2:00 pm

SNACK: Time   **Hours Since Lunch:** Time

I ate/drank:

EAT! Protein

EXERCISE ☐ YES ☐ NO   **TIME** [   ]

What/how much?

_____
_____

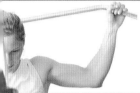

BREATHE IN, BREATHE OUT

When doing resistance exercise, you should **exhale on the exertion** (most difficult part) and **inhale on the recovery** (easiest part). So, when doing an overhead shoulder press for example, you should exhale when you lift the weight over your head, and inhale as you lower it down.

TODAY'S SCHEDULE

3:00 pm

4:00 pm

5:00 pm

DINNER: Time   **Hours Since Snack:** Time

ate/drank:

EAT!

6:00 pm

7:00 pm

8:00 pm

SNACK: Time   **Hours Since Dinner:** Time

ate/drank:

EAT!

9:00 pm

10:00 pm

SNACK: Time   **Hours Since Snack:** Time

ate/drank:

EAT!

11:00 pm

Time I Went to Bed: Time

WATER & EXERCISE

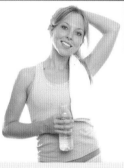

Staying hydrated by drinking water is especially important during exercise. The longer and more intensely you exercise, the more important it becomes for optimal performance. Studies have found that a loss of body fluids due to sweating is linked to a drop in blood volume...and when this occurs, the heart is forced to work harder to move blood through your body. This can lead to muscle cramps, dizziness, fatigue, heat exhaustion and even heat stroke. **Keep your water close by at all times when exercising!**

NOTES

For each 8 oz. glass of water consumed, CIRCLE A NUMBER ➔ 1 2 3 4 5 6 7 8 9 10 11 12

How many hours did you sleep last night? _____

Supplements I took today? _____

You are coming into the home stretch of your *21 Day Metabolism Makeover*! Today, we are going to start to get you prepared for eating in a way that will keep you lean – forever – by making sure you aren't depriving yourself of ANYTHING!

DAY 17: EAT ONLY FOODS YOU LOVE TODAY

Today, you are going to make sure that every single thing you put in your mouth is something that you truly enjoy. If anything you are planning to eat today even vaguely resembles "diet" food – it's off limits today. If your Breakfasts have only been "OK" or your snacks are a bit boring, take the time today to dream up what you'd really "love to have" then find a way to eat those foods on the program.

Focusing On YOUR Favorite Foods

If for some reason you find, at this point in your *21 Day Metabolism Makeover*, that you are eating the same foods or meals over and over again and it's starting to get tiresome -- STOP right now. Don't eat it any more. Don't let the "I have to eat the same boring foods every day to lose weight" diet mentality keep you from enjoying your favorite meals. Be daring and creative! Remember, you MUST be eating foods you LOVE if you want to keep the weight off.

Believe it or not, but you can actually make a Fat Loss Plate that consists of macaroni and cheese, collard greens and pork chops! The majority of people would think macaroni and cheese does not fit the mold when it comes to burning body fat. But most people don't know what you now know which is: that with just a few simple modifications, virtually all of your favorite dishes can be part of a tasty, metabolism-boosting Fat Loss Plate. So, if you are craving a favorite food or dish that you haven't eaten yet – today is a great day to make it part of your Fat Loss Plate.

No More Diets

Many people live their entire lives going from one diet to another. And guess what? They never win at weight loss.

By depriving and restricting themselves of foods they love when on a diet, eventually they give up and go back to their old way of eating – binging on favorite foods – and gaining the weight back and often more.

To make sure you are not "dieting" or depriving yourself and to make sure you are continuing to eat foods you love, ask yourself: "What are my favorite foods and how can I make them a part of a Fat Loss Plate?"

Is It The FOOD or The TASTE You Want?

Many Food Lovers absolutely love to eat deep-fried chicken. Unfortunately, when you submerge chicken in extremely hot grease you not only saturate the chicken with unhealthy fat and cancer-causing Trans Fats, you almost double the calories!

However, Food Lovers don't have to give up fried chicken! In fact, there's another way to eat friend chicken that isn't deep-fried, but tastes like it is. Check out the **Spicy Oven-Fried Chicken** in your *The Love to Eat Cookbook*. The savor and the flavor of deep-fried chicken is exactly what you'll get – not the health-harming and metabolism-slowing effects of the boiling grease that the chicken was submerged in.

With the help of *The Love to Eat Cookbook*, *Classic Comfort Food Recipe Cards*, *Million Meals Menu Planner* and *How to Make a Fat Loss Plate*, you will easily find ways to eat all your favorite foods without hindering your metabolism.

If, for some reason, you aren't able to figure out how to eat your favorite foods without switching your body to "Fat Storing Mode", go to our website (www.MyFoodLovers. com); thanks to the other **Food Lovers** out there, our staff and the constant recipe updates, you can be assured that where there is a will, there is a way to literally have your cake and eat it too.

DO THIS TODAY

1

Eat Only Foods You Love

Today, make sure that every meal and every snack you eat is truly something you enjoy. If you are eating anything that even vaguely resembles diet food, choose something else – *something that you love*. Make a list of your all-time favorite meals, and if you haven't eaten them on the program yet, check over the resources in the program, find out how to tweak them into a Fat Loss Plate and enjoy them today.

2

Get Ready for Tomorrow

Tomorrow, we are going to make the final change to your exercise routine. You are going to upgrade your Fat Burning Cardio to 36 minutes. The *Fight the Fat Kickboxing DVD* is not only a great way to burn A LOT of calories, but it's also a ton of fun. So look over your schedule for tomorrow and make sure you've set aside 36 minutes to accelerate your fat loss with this exuberant and invigorating workout.

DAY 17

EAT ONLY FOODS
YOU LOVE TODAY

Mix up your menu today and leave out anything that isn't exciting and delicious. Make a list of your all-time favorite meals and snacks and find a way to turn them into Food Lovers Meals and Food Lovers Snacks. Don't put anything in your mouth today unless you love it.

✓ TO DO'S
(check when done)

- ☐ Listen to the **Day 17** Audio Program
- ☐ Eat only foods I love today
- ☐ Eat Fat Loss Meals with Accelerator Snacks every 2 to 3 hours
- ☐ Take my nutritional supplements
- ☐ Get 7 to 8 hours of sleep
- ☐ Choose only healthy breads, sweets and fats. Cut back on sodium
- ☐ Drink more water and avoid alcohol
- ☐ _____
- ☐ _____
- ☐ _____
- ☐ _____

TODAY'S CALLS

_____
_____
_____
_____
_____
_____
_____

TODAY'S SCHEDULE

B-FAST / SNACK: Time   **Mins. Since Waking Up:** Time

I ate/drank:

EAT!

7:00 am

8:00 am

9:00 am

B-FAST / SNACK: Time   **Hours Since Breakfast:** Time

I ate/drank:

EAT!

10:00 am

11:00 am

12:00 pm

LUNCH / SNACK: Time   **Hours Since Snack:** Time

I ate/drank:

EAT!

1:00 pm

2:00 pm

SNACK: Time   **Hours Since Lunch:** Time

I ate/drank:

EAT!

EXERCISE ☐ YES ☐ NO   TIME [_____]

What/how much?

_____
_____

LOVE CAKE?

On the **Food Lover Fat Loss System**, you really can have your cake and eat it too. Make sure you check out the Carrot Cake on the *Classic Comfort Food Recipe Cards*. Who knew fat loss could taste so good!

TODAY'S SCHEDULE

3:00 pm

4:00 pm

5:00 pm

DINNER: Time   **Hours Since Snack:** Time

te/drank:

EAT!

6:00 pm

7:00 pm

8:00 pm

SNACK: Time   **Hours Since Dinner:** Time

te/drank:

EAT!

9:00 pm

10:00 pm

SNACK: Time   **Hours Since Snack:** Time

te/drank:

EAT!

11:00 pm

Time I Went to Bed: Time

"Fried" Chicken Wings

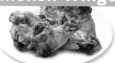

Some Food Lovers crave pizza. Others love a good steak, or pasta, or desserts. The amazing part of Food Lovers is that you don't have to give up your favorite foods. One of our favorite Food Lovers, Brenda, absolutely loves fried chicken wings. Brenda lost more than 100 pounds on the program without giving up her favorite wings. She simply tweaked her recipe to make a great Fat Loss Plate!

"Fried" Chicken Wings
- 1 cup vinegar
- 20 Chicken Wings
- 2 TBSP Smart Balance® Buttery Spread, melted
- Mrs. Dash Garlic Powder to taste
- Pepper to taste
- Non-stick cooking spray

Pre-heat oven broiler to 450 degrees. Fill the kitchen sink half-full of water. Add 1 cup vinegar and soak chicken wings for about 10 minutes. Line a large cookie sheet with aluminum foil and lightly spray with cooking spray. Lay out the wings close together, and brush lightly with Buttery Spread. Season to your taste. Broil for 20 to 30 minutes or until golden brown. Turn wings over and repeat. Remove skin off dark part of meat. Makes 4 servings.

NOTES

For each 8 oz. glass of water consumed, CIRCLE A NUMBER ➔ 1 2 3 4 5 6 7 8 9 10 11 12

w many hours did you sleep last night? _____

pplements I took today? _____

Today you are going to make the final change to your exercise schedule… and have a ton of fun in the process.

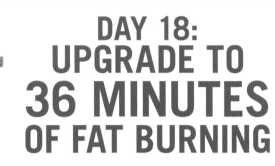

DAY 18:
UPGRADE TO
36 MINUTES
OF FAT BURNING

Starting today and on all your Fat Burning Cardio days going forward, crank it up to 36 minutes. This is as high as you'll need to go to get all the results you want. The simplest way to do this is to pop in your *Fight the Fat Kickboxing DVD*. It has long been the most popular workout because it is terrific fun and will work for virtually any fitness level. If you'd prefer to do some other form of fat burning cardio, just follow the directions for keeping your heart in the "target zone" from Day 8 and keep it there for **36 minutes** continuously.

What's Next?

You are now alternating between 36 minutes of fat burning cardio and 24 minutes of resistance, or "Circuit Training" (the *Tone and Burn DVD*), every other day. This is plenty of weekly exercise to lose all the weight you want and dramatically improve your health and energy levels.

You can continue alternating the two videos for as long as you like. But eventually you'll want to mix it up, to "shock" your body into increasing your fat burning results by doing different exercises as we mentioned on Day 15. This is because after about 3 to 5 weeks of doing the same exercise routine at the same intensity, your body will "adapt" to the exercise and this "adaptation" can slow your weight loss results.

"Adaptation" – Same Workout, Less Results

When you repeat the same activity or exercise routine regularly for a long enough period, your body (muscles) adapts to the stress (demands), and and the activity becomes easier to perform. While this is a real benefit if you are training to run in a marathon, it can be a *liability when it comes to weight loss*. And that's because, as your body adapts and the exercises become easier to do, your body requires less energy to do them. And that means you're burning less calories.

How to Avoid Plateaus

To avoid plateaus that can accompany "adaptation," try to change your workout every 21 days. The **36 Minute Pilates DVD** is a terrific light cardio workout that is also great for the abs, and the **Cardio Funk Fusion DVD** workout is guaranteed to be the most fun you've ever had burning fat.

The other way to avoid "adaptation" plateaus is to incorporate the principles of "Cross Training," which means strategically rotating two or more methods of exercises to maximize results. For example, after you've completed your **21 Day Metabolism Makeover**, try to replace your usual cardio workout with an alternative cardio workout every third time – that's about once every two weeks. If, for instance, you have been walking or doing your **Fight the Fat Kickboxing DVD** for your normal cardio workout, every third time try swimming or going for a bike ride or spending some time on an elliptical machine as an alternative.

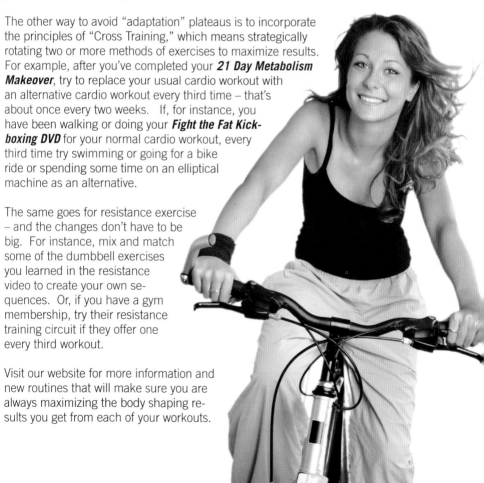

The same goes for resistance exercise – and the changes don't have to be big. For instance, mix and match some of the dumbbell exercises you learned in the resistance video to create your own sequences. Or, if you have a gym membership, try their resistance training circuit if they offer one every third workout.

Visit our website for more information and new routines that will make sure you are always maximizing the body shaping results you get from each of your workouts.

DAY 18

Optimizing Your Eating Schedule Round II

You learned how to adjust your eating schedule on the days you are working out back on Day 12. As a reminder, the charts below will give you some real-world examples of what ideal eating schedules look like depending on what time of day you like to do your workout.

Always Eat a Meal Within 1 Hour of Working Out

MORNING WORKOUT (*NO SNACK*)*

If you are only doing LIGHT cardio (like the *12 Minute Fat Burning Cardio DVD* or a low-intensity "fun" fat burning activity like walking), you can skip snacking before your workout if you aren't ready to eat first thing in the morning and simply begin the day with your workout. Just make sure to eat a FULL Breakfast ("Post-Workout Meal") within 60 minutes (ideally 30 minutes) of completing your workout.

YOUR DAILY TIMELINE	
WAKE UP	5:15 AM
Begin Workout	5:45 AM
Complete Workout	6:15 AM
Breakfast	6:45 AM
Snack	9:30 AM
Lunch	11:30 AM
Snack	2:30 PM
Snack	5:00 PM
Dinner	7:30 PM
SLEEP	10:00 PM

MORNING WORKOUT (*WITH SNACK*)

If you are doing high-intensity cardio like today's 36 minute video or ANY resistance workout, you MUST have a snack BEFORE your workout. Then eat a FULL Breakfast ("Post-Workout Meal") within 60 minutes (ideally 30 minutes) of completing your workout.

YOUR DAILY TIMELINE	
WAKE UP	5:15 AM
Snack	5:45 AM
Begin Workout	6:30 AM
Complete Workout	7:15 AM
Breakfast	8:00 AM
Snack	10:30 AM
Lunch	1:00 PM
Snack	3:30 PM
Dinner	6:00 PM
Snack	8:00 PM
SLEEP	11:30 PM

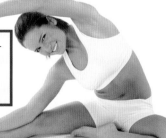

*Note: If you tend to get panicky, angry or lightheaded after going long periods without eating, you may tend towards "hypoglycemia" and should always eat a snack or meal BEFORE any workout.

AFTERNOON WORKOUT

The following chart shows a typical workout schedule for those who like to work out after work. Here you would have two afternoon snacks to provide energy for your workout, then Dinner ("Post-Workout Meal") within 60 minutes of finishing the workout.

YOUR DAILY TIMELINE

WAKE UP	8:30 AM
Breakfast	9:15 AM
Lunch	12:00 PM
Snack	2:00 PM
Snack	4:30 PM
Begin Workout	5:30 PM
Complete Workout	6:15 PM
Dinner	7:00 PM
Snack	9:30 PM
SLEEP	11:30 PM

NIGHTTIME WORKOUT

For those who like to work out after Dinner, the schedule looks a bit different. Since you ALWAYS eat a meal after a workout, you have two choices: (1) at around 6:00 p.m. when you would normally have dinner, you could choose another snack instead, then workout and have a full Fat Loss Meal after your workout -- around 8:30 or 9:00. Or (2), as shown in this example, if you still want to have Dinner with your family at 6:00 p.m. you could actually add a fourth meal to your day. For best results, at 6:00 choose a Version B Fat Loss Plate (more **Slow Carb** and no **Fast Carb**). Then after your workout have a normal Fat Loss Meal.

YOUR DAILY TIMELINE

WAKE UP	7:00 AM
Breakfast	7:30 AM
Snack	10:00 AM
Lunch	12:30 PM
Snack	3:30 PM
Dinner (Version B)	6:00 PM
Begin Workout	7:00 PM
Complete Workout	7:45 PM
Dinner (4th Meal)	8:30 PM
SLEEP	11:00 PM

DO THIS TODAY

1 **Upgrade to 36 Minutes of Fat Burning**
Starting today, increase your fat burning workouts to 36 minutes. The simplest way is to pop in the *Fight the Fat Kickboxing DVD*. It's fun and incredibly effective.

2 **Get Ready for Tomorrow**
Tomorrow, you are going to learn how to spot hidden "calorie bombs" in all your meals and snacks. You'll do that by making sure you know the nutritional breakdown of everything you eat tomorrow. So, if you are planning to eat out at a restaurant for any meal tomorrow, try to get nutritional information from them today so you can look it over before you go. Many national chains will provide it online or call the restaurant to see if they have that info they can fax you.

DAY 18

UPGRADE TO 36 MINUTES
OF FAT BURNING

Starting today, increase your fat burning workouts to 36 minutes
The simplest way is to pop in your *Fight the Fat Kickboxing DVD*.
fun and incredibly effective.

TO DO'S
(check when done)

- [ ] Listen to the **Day 18** Audio Program
- [ ] Do 36 mins of fat burning cardio
- [ ] Eat Fat Loss Meals with Accelerator Snacks every 2 to 3 hours
- [ ] Take my nutritional supplements
- [ ] Get 7 to 8 hours of sleep
- [ ] Choose only healthy breads, sweets and fats. Cut back on sodium
- [ ] Drink more water and avoid alcohol
- [ ] _____
- [ ] _____
- [ ] _____
- [ ] _____

TODAY'S CALLS

_____
_____
_____
_____
_____
_____
_____
_____

TODAY'S SCHEDULE

B-FAST / SNACK: Time   **Mins. Since Waking Up:** Time

I ate/drank:

EAT! Protein

7:00 am

8:00 am

9:00 am

B-FAST / SNACK: Time   **Hours Since Breakfast:** Time

I ate/drank:

EAT! Protein

10:00 am

11:00 am

12:00 pm

LUNCH / SNACK: Time   **Hours Since Snack:** Time

I ate/drank:

EAT! Protein

1:00 pm

2:00 pm

SNACK: Time   **Hours Since Lunch:** Time

I ate/drank:

EAT! Protein

EXERCISE ☐ YES ☐ NO   TIME

What/how much?

PRE-EXERCISE FUEL

Morning workouts are great, but it is important to put some fuel into your body to get thru the workout. Here's the easy recipe for a delicious Berry-Berry Banana Smoothie: 1/2 cup frozen blueberries, 1/2 Banana, 1 scoop of Protein Powder and water blended until frosty-smooth. This snack is a tasty way to give your body the fuel it needs to power thru your workout!

TODAY'S SCHEDULE

:00 pm _____

:00 pm _____

:00 pm _____

NNER: Time   **Hours Since Snack:** Time

te/drank: _____

EAT! _____
_____

:00 pm _____

:00 pm _____

:00 pm _____

NACK: Time   **Hours Since Dinner:** Time

te/drank: _____

EAT! _____
_____

:00 pm _____

:00 pm _____

NACK: Time   **Hours Since Snack:** Time

te/drank: _____

EAT! _____
_____

:00 pm _____
_____

Time I Went to Bed: Time

EATING & EXERCISING - OPTIMIZING THE SCHEDULE

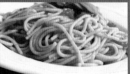

As we've said many times, for fast fat loss results it is of critical importance that you NEVER let more than 3 hours elapse without eating. This becomes even more important as you add more intense exercise to your schedule.

Even though the workouts you are doing are relatively brief, they are extremely efficient and will very quickly burn through the blood sugar that supplies you with energy. Because of this, you need to make sure you are eating enough food to provide sufficient energy to perform your workouts and to prevent your blood sugar levels from dropping too drastically; if this occurs, it can sap your energy and cause uncontrollable hunger.

NOTES

For each 8 oz. glass of water consumed, **CIRCLE A NUMBER** ➔ 1 2 3 4 5 6 7 8 9 10 11 12

w many hours did you sleep last night? _____

pplements I took today? _____

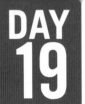

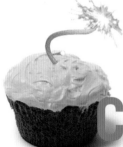

DAY 19: LEARN TO AVOID HIDDEN CALORIE BOMBS

Today, you are going to apply everything you've learned so far about food and how it affects your metabolism and read – and understand – the nutritional labels on every single thing you eat. **When you cook a meal, carefully go over the labels and read every ingredient, and do the same with every snack. If you go out to eat, have the restaurant supply nutritional information, if available**. Pay attention to the total calories in the foods you prepare or order, take notice of small things with unusually high calorie counts, compare percentages and types of fat, notice how much protein and carbohydrates – especially sugar – are in foods. Pay attention to the sodium content and the amount of fiber.

From the time you wake up to the time you go to bed, make sure you understand the nutritional makeup of everything you put in your body. That's it. That's all you have to do today. You can then choose to eat it or not, it's up to you. Today is just about understanding what is in your food and being more aware of exactly what you are putting in your body. After that, it's up to you.

Calories and the Fat Loss Program

On the **Food Lovers Fat Loss System** you don't count calories, fat grams or anything else. The way the program is designed, you don't have to. The portions and combination of the Fat Loss Plate automatically control your calorie intake. But, just because you don't have to count them, doesn't mean calories don't matter.

No matter how fast you get your metabolism going, if you consume more calories than your now-racing metabolism can use, your body is going to have no choice but to store the unused surplus as fat. And some foods actually pack so many calories into such tiny packages that you can inadvertently slow your weight loss. Today we're going to focus on how to avoid these calorie "bombs."

Calorie "Bombs"

When you've tried to lose weight in the past, how often did you opt for a salad because you thought it would help you lose weight? Did you know that a Caesar Salad can easily contain more than 800 calories and 30 grams of fat!

Unfortunately, tremendous amounts of calories can lurk in sauces, dressings, restaurant foods and all sorts of pre-packaged products – even "healthy" looking products – waiting to sabotage your weight loss goals. Particularly when it comes to dining out and eating packaged foods (including snacks), you really need to KNOW what it is you are eating. Because of the way food is packaged, marketed and prepared these days, if you aren't diligent, these pre-packaged foods and restaurant meals could seriously affect your fat loss efforts. So while the ultimate goal is to lose fat while still enjoying your favorite foods without having to count calories, it pays to be aware of the caloric content of the foods, drinks and condiments you consume and act accordingly. Fortunately, nutrition labels can be a big help.

JENNIFER'S STORY

Lost 50 lbs
On the Food Lovers Fat Loss System

BEFORE **AFTER**

Jennife thought she was doing everything she could to reduce her waistline by making sure every meal was a proper Fat Loss Plate. Little did she know, the restaurants she was visiting were inadvertently sabotaging her weight loss results.

She frequented a family restaurant chain and dutifully ordered a Fat Loss Plate: a baked dish of white-meat chicken (**Protein**), penne pasta (**Fast Carb**), and broccoli (**Slow Carb**). The proportions were right and, even though the pasta was tossed in a parmesan cream sauce and topped with cheddar cheese, Jennifer asked that the sauce be applied lightly with only a light sprinkle of cheese for flavor.

After many visits, Jennifer asked if she could get a "Nutritional Fact Sheet" which breaks down the nutritional info for each item on the menu (practically all major restaurant chains provide them). Since she was a regular patron of the restaurant, she thought it would be valuable to get a sense of where the calories really lurked on the menu.

To Jennifer's surprise, her perfect Fat Loss Plate actually contained **2,060 calories and 128 grams of fat!** But, after reviewing the nutritional info the restaurant provided, she found many other dishes that she loved, (even preferred), some that she wrongly assumed would be "off limits," that were indeed great choices for weight loss. Having honed her Label Detective skills, Jennifer went on to lose 50 pounds with even MORE great tasting choices at her favorite restaurants.

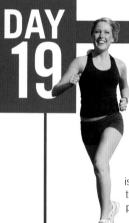

WHAT IS A CALORIE?

Most people think a calorie is something that makes you fat – perhaps a measurement of how fattening a food is. The fact of the matter is, a calorie is a measurement of energy. That's right. The higher the calories in a food, the more potential energy it contains. The energy stored in food, is measured in terms of calories.

Technically, one calorie is the amount of energy required to raise the temperature of one gram of water one degree Centigrade. The calorie measure used commonly to discuss the energy content of food is actually a kilocalorie (Kcal), which equals 1000 real calories. This is the amount of energy required to raise one kilogram of water (about 2.2 pounds) one degree Centigrade.

Decoding Nutrition Labels

Look before you lunch! Scan before you snack! Get in the habit of checking out a food's nutrition facts box before you start scarfing it up.

Food companies are actually required by law to give you the plain facts about what you're about to eat. But since no food company will ever say something like, "This food is bad for you! Choose something healthier!", it takes some practice to read these labels and know what you're looking at.

UNDERSTANDING FOOD LABELS

A CLOSER LOOK AT THE LABEL

Serving Size: 1 oz. Located at the top of the label, this tells you the amount of food used to measure all the other numbers on the label. The serving size for this food (cheese crunchies) is 1 ounce, which equals about 21 cheese crunchies.

Servings Per Container: About 2. This tells you how many servings are in the bag. In this case, it says "about 2," but since the serving size is 1 ounce, and the bag contains over 2 ounces, a little math will tell you that there are really MORE than two servings in the bag. Okay, so what does it mean? Well, since most people will eat the whole bag of snacks (it's a small bag, after all) and the numbers listed only apply to one ounce (half the bag), that means you're really getting TWICE as much as the label says! So if the label says 170 calories per serving, and you eat the whole bag (2 servings), you're really eating 340 calories!

Remember: A lot of food companies will make their food "serving size" small, so it looks like the food is healthier than it really is and you may be surprised what they consider a serving. It may actually be only HALF a blueberry muffin or 10 or 12 nuts in a bag of 100 nuts, so make sure you always look at how many servings are in a bag, box, or can of food BEFORE you look at the rest of the numbers. Depending on how much of the food you eat, you may have to double or triple the other numbers on the label.

Nutrition Facts

Serving Size 1 oz. (28g/about 21 pieces)
Servings Per Container About 2

Amount per serving

Calories 170	Calories from Fat 110

	% Daily Value*
Tatal Fat 11g	**17%**
Saturated Fat 1.5g	**8%**
Trans Fat 0 g	
Cholesterol 0 g	**0%**
Sodium 250mg	**10%**
Total Carbohydrate 14g	**5%**
Dietary Fiber less than 1g	**2%**
Sugars 0g	
Protein 2g	

Vitamin A 2%	*	Vitamin C 0%
Calcium 0%	*	Iron 4%
Vitamin E 6%	*	Thiamin 4%
Riboflavin 2%	*	Niacin 4%
Vitamin B6 2%	*	Phosphorus 2%

*Percent Daily Values are based on a 2,000 calorie diet. Your daily values may be higher or lower depending on your calorie needs:

		Calories:	2,000	2,500
Total Fat	Less than		65g	80g
Sat Fat	Less than		20g	25g
Cholesterol	Less than		300mg	300mg
Sodium	Less than		2,400mg	2,400mg
Total Carbohydrate			300g	375g
Dietary Fiber			25g	30g

Calories per gram:
Fat 9   *   Carbohydrate 4   *   Protein 4

NUTRITIONAL BREAKDOWN
OF A FAT LOSS PLATE

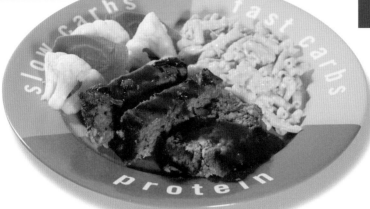

On **Food Lovers** you don't have to count calories, fat grams or anything else. The portions of a Fat Loss plate, combined with your knowledge of how to avoid the biggest "Enemies of Fat Loss," does that automatically. But since we're all about reading labels today, imagine that a typical Fat Loss Plate you make at home came with a nutritional label -- what would that look like?

Obviously, a Fat Loss Plate will vary from meal to meal, depending on a variety of factors but, in general, a well made Fat Loss Plate will end up with the following approximate breakdown:

	MEN	WOMEN
Total Calories	300 - 550 (Never more than 600)	250 - 450 (Never more than 500)
Protein	15g - 40g	15g - 30g
Carbohydrates	30g - 50g	30g - 45g
Fat	20 - 30% or LESS of total calories	20 - 30% or LESS of total calories
Fiber	At least 5g (30 - 38g /day)	At least 5g (20 - 25g /day)
Sodium	LESS than 700 mgs	LESS than 700 mgs

DO THIS TODAY

1

Learn To Avoid Hidden "Calorie Bombs"

For today, read – and UNDERSTAND – the nutritional information associated with everything you eat, cook or order at a restaurant. It will help you truly understand where the hidden "calorie bombs" are in your food – so you can concentrate on other foods that you love that will help, rather than hinder, your fat loss efforts.

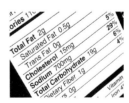

DAY 19

LEARN TO AVOID HIDDEN
CALORIE BOMBS

Today, read and understand the nutritional makeup of everything you eat. Whether you eat it or not is up to you. The key today is to get a sense of when the calories and hidden "Enemies of Fat Loss" lurk in the foods you e

✓ TO DO'S
(check when done)

- ☐ Listen to the **Day 19** Audio Program
- ☐ Read nutritional info on everything I eat today
- ☐ Eat Fat Loss Meals with Accelerator Snacks every 2 to 3 hours
- ☐ Take my nutritional supplements
- ☐ Get 7 to 8 hours of sleep
- ☐ Choose only healthy breads, sweets and fats. Cut back on sodium.
- ☐ Drink more water and avoid alcohol
- ☐ _____
- ☐ _____
- ☐ _____
- ☐ _____

TODAY'S CALLS

_____
_____
_____
_____
_____
_____
_____

TODAY'S SCHEDULE

B-FAST / SNACK: Time   **Mins. Since Waking Up:** Time

I ate/drank:

EAT!
_____
_____

7:00 am _____

8:00 am _____

9:00 am _____

B-FAST / SNACK: Time   **Hours Since Breakfast:** Time

I ate/drank:

EAT!
_____
_____

10:00 am _____

11:00 am _____

12:00 pm _____

LUNCH / SNACK: Time   **Hours Since Snack:** Time

I ate/drank:

EAT!
_____
_____

1:00 pm _____

2:00 pm _____

SNACK: Time   Lunch   **Hours Since Lunch:** Time

I ate/drank:

EAT!
_____
_____

EXERCISE   ☐ YES   ☐ NO   TIME [_____]

What/how much?
_____
_____

SMALL BITES, LARGE CALORIE COUNT

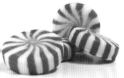

You know those little mints at the restaurant that you nibble on while waiting to get seated OR your server gives them to you with your bill? Well, 3 of those are about 90 calories – serving size is 5 which is about 147 calories. Yikes! That's a whole snack in one bite!

TODAY'S SCHEDULE

:00 pm _____

:00 pm _____

:00 pm _____

NNER: Time _____ Hours Since Snack: Time

te/drank: _____

EAT!

:00 pm _____

:00 pm _____

:00 pm _____

NACK: Time _____ Hours Since Dinner: Time

te/drank: _____

EAT!

:00 pm _____

:00 pm _____

NACK: Time _____ Hours Since Snack: Time

te/drank: _____

EAT!

:00 pm _____

Time I Went to Bed: Time

CALORIES FROM FAT

Which Would You Choose?

Med. French Fries
380 Calories

OR

Turkey & Gravy Dinner
(Classic Comfort Foods Recipe)
380 Calories

12 Tortilla Chips
200 Calories

OR

Soft Taco & Black Beans
(Classic Comfort Foods Recipe)
200 Calories

NOTES

For each 8 oz. glass of water consumed, CIRCLE A NUMBER ➜ 1 2 3 4 5 6 7 8 9 10 11 12

ow many hours did you sleep last night? _____

upplements I took today? _____

By now *you are truly an expert on food, nutrition and weight loss*. You know more about eating in a way that will cause you to lose weight than most trainers and nutritionists at gyms – perhaps even your doctor – and now it's time to share your knowledge. This will not only give you the opportunity to help a friend but will reinforce your knowledge and make it easier to **keep the weight off... forever**.

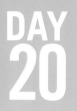

DAY 20: SERVE A
FAT LOSS MEAL
TO A FRIEND

Today, you are going to prepare and serve a Fat Loss Plate to a friend. **Choose one of your favorite meals, something that could never be confused with diet food, and without telling your friend it is food from your plan, sit down and enjoy the meal**. Then afterwards, tell him / her your secret.

Your Fat Loss Secret

Over the last three weeks, some of your friends have probably already noticed that you are eating differently, and you've probably received a variety of reactions. Some folks may have noticed that you are snacking on delicious treats between meals and may have incorrectly guessed that, since you are "eating all the time," you must have given up your weight loss efforts and simply thrown caution to the wind.

Others may have noticed that you are looking leaner and have much more energy and assume that you've either gone on a crash "diet" or started to kill yourself with exercise. And even if you've explained the program to him/her in detail, chances are they still don't understand it, or even more likely, don't believe it.

That's because almost no one knows the basic truth about weight loss that you now know: **That most people make losing weight much harder than it needs to be**. *They think that suffering and deprivation are required for results.* And, for many, until they see – and taste – for themselves what you're eating, they won't be able to believe how easy – and delicious – being lean and healthy can really be. **Today you are going to share your knowledge – and help a friend**.

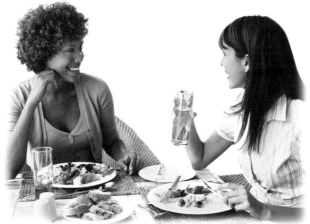

Invite a Friend Over

You can invite anyone you want as long as they don't live with you. Perhaps you know someone who has been struggling with his/her weight over the years, suffering and depriving themselves unnecessarily. Perhaps it is a skeptic who believes that any weight loss plan that claims to allow you to still eat your favorite foods is a bunch of "marketing hooey." Or maybe it is a "foodie" friend who doesn't believe that healthy food prepared and served in a way that will accelerate your metabolism could ever truly be tasty.

Whoever you invite, make sure it is someone you like to spend time with and keep it very casual. Don't tell them why you are inviting them over. Find another excuse to get together and offer to make lunch or dinner… or even breakfast. Maybe invite another parent to bring the kids over to discuss school or have a play-date and prepare a simple supper. You can even tell them you want to try a new recipe you found – just don't tell them it's a Fat Loss Meal.

Choose Your Menu

Keep it simple. Make something that you've made before over the last few weeks – something your family really liked. If you're insecure about your cooking skills or you've fallen into a rut where you are eating the same dish over and over, this is another opportunity to expand your horizons a bit.

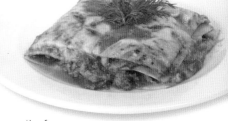

Try something new, or think of something you used to love before you started the program. Then use **The Love to Eat Cookbook** or **Classic Comfort Food Recipe Cards** to learn how to turn it into a Fat Loss Meal. It doesn't need to be fancy. It just needs to taste good. Simple comfort foods like the ones you ate as a kid – lasagna, pot roast, or meatloaf and mashed potatoes – are the foods people tend to love the best and the ones they generally think are impossible to eat in a way that will cause them to lose weight.

Mum's the Word

Here's the key to this day's activity: **Don't say anything about the program or what you are cooking until AFTER dinner**. Don't tell your friend that the meal you are serving them will accelerate their metabolism and help them lose weight. Just serve the meal and enjoy each other's company.

Then Reveal Your Secret...

Once you've both finished the meal, wait ten or fifteen minutes then reveal your secret. Tell your friend that the meal they just ate had just the right combination of foods prepared in a way that switches the body from "Fat Storing Mode" to "Fat Burning Mode." Explain the concept of the Fat Loss Plate and how, by making just a few simple tweaks, you can turn any meal into a Fat Loss Meal. Tell them how you snack BETWEEN meals and into the evening to speed up your metabolism.

Tell them all about the program… and then tell them how you "feel." How your energy has increased… How your clothes are fitting more loosely… How easy it really is!

By sharing what you've learned over the last three weeks, you are not only helping a friend, you are reinforcing everything that you've learned about food and how your metabolism works which will help you stay lean and healthy for the rest of your life.

And if you are still talking a couple hours later, serve them a sweet Food Lovers Snack for dessert!

One of the best ways to truly understand something that you, yourself, have learned is to teach it to someone else. And that is the point of today's exercise.

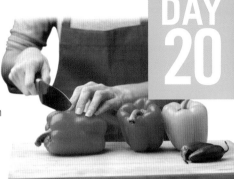

DO THIS TODAY

DAY 20

Serve a Fat Loss Meal to a Friend

Invite someone to come to your house and make and serve him/her a Fat Loss Plate. Don't tell them it is a Fat Loss Plate until **after** you've eaten; then tell them your secret. Explain the program and share your results.

Redo Your Self-Assessment

You are almost done with your *21 Day Metabolism Makeover*. Tomorrow you will get back on the scale, re-take all your body measurements and find out how your body has **actually** changed in the last 3 weeks. But keep in mind, while consciously you embarked on this program to **look** better, if you are being totally honest with yourself, what you really wanted was to **feel** better about yourself -- to feel more attractive, healthy and, at the end of the day, happy. So today, before you take your body measurements, go back to page 15 of the *Rapid Results Success Journal* and redo your Self-Assessment to see how you feel about your body and your health after less than 3 weeks on the **Food Lovers Fat Loss System**.

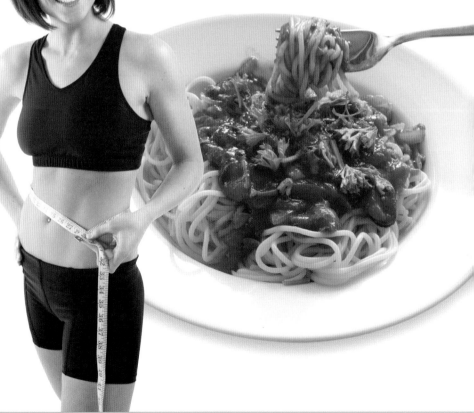

DAY 20

SERVE A FAT LOSS MEAL
TO A FRIEND

Invite a friend to come over and serve them a Fat Loss Plate.
Don't tell them it's a meal that will cause them to lose weight
until after you've eaten. Then explain the program to them.

✓ TO DO'S
(check when done)

- [ ] Listen to the **Day 20** Audio Program
- [ ] Serve a Fat Loss Plate to a friend
- [ ] Eat Fat Loss Meals with Accelerator Snacks every 2 to 3 hours
- [ ] Take my nutritional supplements
- [ ] Get 7 to 8 hours of sleep
- [ ] Choose only healthy breads, sweets and fats. Cut back on sodium
- [ ] Drink more water and avoid alcohol
- [ ] _____
- [ ] _____
- [ ] _____
- [ ] _____

TODAY'S CALLS

_____
_____
_____
_____
_____
_____

TODAY'S SCHEDULE

B-FAST / SNACK: Time   **Mins. Since Waking Up:** Time

I ate/drank:

EAT!

7:00 am

8:00 am

9:00 am

B-FAST / SNACK: Time   **Hours Since Breakfast:** Time

I ate/drank:

EAT!

10:00 am

11:00 am

12:00 pm

LUNCH / SNACK: Time   **Hours Since Snack:** Time

I ate/drank:

EAT!

1:00 pm

2:00 pm

SNACK: Time   Lunch   **Hours Since Lunch:** Time

I ate/drank:

EAT!

EXERCISE   ☐ YES   ☐ NO   TIME ☐

What/how much?

_____
_____

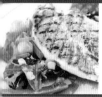

PRESENTATION IS KEY

A Chinese proverb says, "A good meal is eaten first with the eyes, then with the nose and finally with the mouth. Satisfy these and the stomach will rejoice." Take the extra step in making your meals look as great as they taste!

TODAY'S SCHEDULE

:00 pm _____

:00 pm _____

:00 pm _____

NNER: Time   **Hours Since Snack:** Time

e/drank: _____

AT! _____

:00 pm _____

:00 pm _____

:00 pm _____

ACK: Time   **Hours Since Dinner:** Time

e/drank: _____

AT! _____

:00 pm _____

:00 pm _____

ACK: Time   **Hours Since Snack:** Time

e/drank: _____

AT! _____

:00 pm _____

_____

Time I Went to Bed: Time

AMERICA'S FAVORITE FOODS

SOUTHERN FRIED CHICKEN

MACARONI AND CHEESE

JOE'S HOMEMADE CHILI

MOM'S APPLE PIE

A recent article listed the Top 16 foods Americans love most...and nearly half of them are in the *Classic Comfort Food Recipe Cards*. From Fried Chicken to Macaroni & Cheese to Chili to good ol' Apple Pie -- whether cooking for yourself or a guest, you can't go wrong with these scrumptious recipes!

NOTES

For each 8 oz. glass of water consumed, **CIRCLE A NUMBER** ➜ 1 2 3 4 5 6 7 8 9 10 11 12

w many hours did you sleep last night? _____

pplements I took today? _____

Congratulations. **You've done it**. You have reset your metabolism and turned your body into a fat burning machine. Over the next few weeks you are going to see very dramatic results but for today, it's time to celebrate!

DAY 21:
MEASURE... AND CELEBRATE...
YOUR SUCCESS!

Today you'll finish your **21 Day Metabolism Makeover** by assessing your results. Open the **Rapid Results Success Journal**, take all your measurements again then re-calculate your Body Composition Analysis to determine your current Body Fat Percentage. Congratulations! Whether you've lost a little or a lot, you have successfully reset your metabolism. And that means you are ready to move to the next phase, **Food Lovers for Life**, where you'll integrate all your favorite foods into your lifestyle without ever having to worry about gaining weight again.

Okay, You Can Step on the Scale Now...

We know you've been waiting anxiously for this day. You've done everything that's been asked of you – done everything you needed to do to ramp up your metabolism to the point where you are burning calories at a tremendous rate. Now it's time to check out the results.

Start by re-taking all the measurements that you took three weeks ago and record them all in the Measurement Chart in the **Rapid Results Success Journal**. Then step on the scale and redo your Body Composition Analysis to determine your current Body Fat Percentage.

Evaluate Progress

Now it's time to evaluate your progress. Most people start by looking at their change in body weight. And if you've lost a lot of pounds, congratulations! It is not uncommon for people to lose significant amounts of weight in just the first few weeks on this program. But make sure to be realistic. Everyone drops pounds at different rates (men generally lose faster than women). More importantly, please keep in mind that body weight is NOT the best way to measure your success.

Your REAL Results

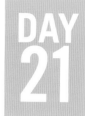

Take a moment and remind yourself why you started this program. It wasn't to reach a certain number on the scale – no one ever sees that number but you. No, you started the program because you wanted to LOOK better and FEEL better. You wanted to fit into smaller clothes, be more attractive and more healthy… *and the scale can't measure any of those things.*

The two most accurate ways to measure your success are with inches and Body Fat Percentage. So look very closely at these numbers. You are now eating and exercising in a way that helps preserve and build lean muscle tissue. Having more lean muscle tissue is not only the key to burning fat… it looks good too.

The thing that is important to remember is that muscle weighs MORE than fat (a pound of muscle takes up 5 times LESS space on your waist than a pound of fat). It is very common for people to lose large amounts of body fat and a significant number of inches while their weight stays basically the same. So don't let the results from the scale be the sole measure of your success.

You got into this to lose FAT and that will be reflected most accurately in lost inches and in Body Fat Percentage. So, no matter what the scale says, **these measurements will reveal your real success**. Compare them to your starting measurements and see just how far you've come in only 21 days!

Celebrate Your Success

You've reached the first landmark. In fact, you've done the hardest part of the program and whether you've lost just a few inches or a whole lot of inches, you have successfully *reset* your metabolism. It is now burning fat faster than ever and over the coming weeks you will see even more dramatic results!* Now it's time to celebrate your success.

Flip back through the Goal Setting Section of the **Rapid Results Success Journal** (Pages 26 to 31) and treat yourself to whatever "Reward" you gave yourself in that section. Whether it's a day at the spa, a new pair of jeans or an evening out – you deserve it. You have accomplished something in the last 3 weeks that will literally change your life forever! So mark the occasion with something that's "just for you."

*(NOTE: If you still feel you aren't seeing results as quickly as you should be, read over the Troubleshooting Guide on pages 34 to 35 of the **Rapid Results Success Journal** and just keep eating the way you've been shown. Everyone's metabolism kicks in at a different point on the program, and when it does, the fat begins to melt off very rapidly. If you continue to follow the tenets of **Food Lovers**, it is impossible to fail!)*

DAY 21

BRETT'S STORY

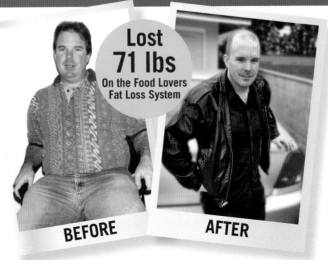

Lost 71 lbs
On the Food Lovers Fat Loss System

BEFORE   **AFTER**

On the day Brett started the *21 Day Metabolism Makeover* he weighed 256 pounds. He was excited and motivated and followed the plan to a "T." He made sure to eat every 3 hours and to combine his meals into Fat Loss Plates. He conscientiously chose healthy fats, breads and sweets and kept a vigilant watch for the biggest enemies of fat loss. He even found a way to make sure he was getting more sleep.

By the end of 21 days he felt great. He had more energy, a better attitude and he could feel that his clothes were looser. He felt stronger and leaner and just knew he had done "pretty darn well"… until he stepped on the scale. On the morning of the 21st day, Brett stepped on the scale again and it read: 256 pounds - exactly the same weight as when he started.

Naturally, his first impulse was to be discouraged. And then he looked a bit more closely at his results. He took new measurements of his body and redid his Body Composition Analysis and things started to look a little different.

When Brett started the *21 Day Metabolism Makeover* his body fat percentage was 34%. That meant that 87.04 pounds of his weight was fat and he had an LBM (Lean Body Mass) of 168.96 pounds. Now, when he recalculated his Body Fat Percentage, it was down to 31.9 percent. That meant his "fat" weight had dropped from 87.04 pounds to 81.6 pounds. **That's a Fat Loss of 5.37 pounds… in just 3 weeks!***

What Brett hadn't realized was that while he was losing fat, he had gained 5.3 pounds of lean body mass, which caused his total body weight to remain the same. And since he replaced the fat with lean muscle tissue he had increased his fat burning potential. Since he has more lean body mass he is burning more calories all day long.

Brett had truly reset his metabolism and turned his body into a fat burning machine - which meant every time he recalculated his results he would lose weight at a faster rate. In fact, **he went on to reach his goal, losing 71 pounds and he's now living life a lean, healthy 185 pounds**.

*[0.5 – 1 percent body reduction in 21 days is great. 1.5 or higher in 21 days is absolutely phenomenal

Tomorrow...

Your metabolism should now be racing and tomorrow you move into the next phase of the program where you learn to integrate EVERY single one of your favorite foods back into your everyday life and still lose all the weight you want. Plus you'll learn how to stay lean and healthy for the rest of your life. You've already done the hard part. The rest is easy!

DO THIS TODAY

1 **Measure... and Celebrate... Your Success!**

Retake all your measurements, weigh yourself and record it all in the *Rapid Results Success Journal*. Then recalculate your Body Composition Analysis to determine your fat loss over the last 21 days. Then celebrate your success with whatever reward you promised yourself in the *Rapid Results Success Journal*.

2 **Get Ready For Tomorrow**

You've finished the most difficult part of the program. Tomorrow you start the *Food Lovers for Life* program where you'll learn how to integrate all of your favorite foods into your life so you can stay lean and healthy forever. Sometime today or early tomorrow morning, listen to Week 1 on the *Food Lovers for Life CD*. Swap out this *21 Metabolism Makeover* book for the *Food Lovers for Life* book and get ready to lose all the weight you want and be lean and healthy for the rest of your life.

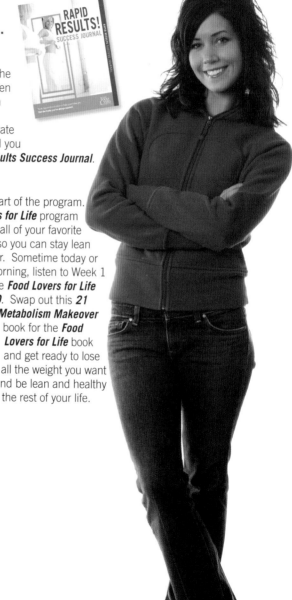

DAY 21

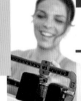

MEASURE... AND CELEBRATE...
YOUR SUCCESS

Retake all your measurements, weigh yourself, and record it all in your **Rapid Results Success Journal**. Then retake your Body Composition Analysis and celebrate your success with the reward you promised yourself in your **Rapid Results Success Journal**.

✓ TO DO'S
(check when done)

- ☐ Listen to the **Day 21** Audio Program
- ☐ Retake all measurements for **Rapid Results** and enjoy your reward!
- ☐ Eat Fat Loss Meals with Accelerator Snacks every 2 to 3 hours
- ☐ Take my nutritional supplements
- ☐ Get 7 to 8 hours of sleep
- ☐ Choose only healthy breads, sweets and fats. Cut back on sodium
- ☐ Drink more water and avoid alcohol
- ☐ _____
- ☐ _____
- ☐ _____

TODAY'S CALLS

_____
_____
_____
_____
_____
_____
_____
_____

TODAY'S SCHEDULE

B-FAST / SNACK: Time   **Mins. Since Waking Up:** Time

I ate/drank:

EAT!

7:00 am

8:00 am

9:00 am

B-FAST / SNACK: Time   **Hours Since Breakfast:** Time

I ate/drank:

EAT!

10:00 am

11:00 am

12:00 pm

LUNCH / SNACK: Time   **Hours Since Snack:** Time

I ate/drank:

EAT!

1:00 pm

2:00 pm

SNACK: Time   Lunch   **Hours Since Lunch:** Time

I ate/drank:

EAT!

EXERCISE ☐ YES ☐ NO   TIME

What/how much?

_____
_____

CONGRATULATIONS!

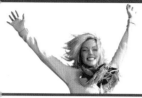

You have reset your metabolism so you are now burning fat at a tremendous rate. You've learned how to eat in a way that will cause you to lose all the weight you want and be lean and healthy for the rest of your life!

TODAY'S SCHEDULE

3:00 pm

4:00 pm

5:00 pm

DINNER: Time   **Hours Since Snack:** Time

ate/drank:

EAT!

6:00 pm

7:00 pm

8:00 pm

SNACK: Time   **Hours Since Dinner:** Time

ate/drank:

EAT!

9:00 pm

10:00 pm

SNACK: Time   **Hours Since Snack:** Time

ate/drank:

EAT!

11:00 pm

Time I Went to Bed: Time

REWARD YOURSELF FOR MAKING IT TO DAY 21

A day at the spa?

A new outfit?

Champagne and a chocolate-dipped strawberry?

MAKE YOUR REWARD EXTRA SPECIAL!

NOTES:

For each 8 oz. glass of water consumed, CIRCLE A NUMBER ➔ 1 2 3 4 5 6 7 8 9 10 11 12

How many hours did you sleep last night? _____

Supplements I took today? _____

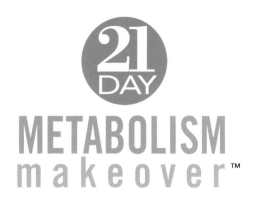

Congratulations!

You've completed your *21 Day Metabolism Makeover*! It's now time to begin *Food Lovers for Life*, so take this book out of your binder and insert the *Food Lovers for Life* book. Take the time now to read the Introduction and Week 1 sections of *Food Lovers for Life*.